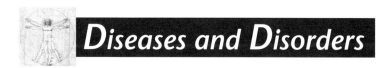

Acne

by Barbara Sheen

LUCENT
BOOKS®

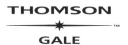

THOMSON
— ✦ —™
GALE

San Diego • Detroit • New York • San Francisco • Cleveland
New Haven, Conn. • Waterville, Maine • London • Munich

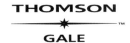
THOMSON
GALE

© 2004 by Lucent Books. Lucent Books is an imprint of The Gale Group, Inc.,
a division of Thomson Learning, Inc.

Lucent Books® and Thomson Learning™ are trademarks used herein under license.

For more information, contact
Lucent Books
27500 Drake Rd.
Farmington Hills, MI 48331-3535
Or you can visit our Internet site at http://www.gale.com

LIBRARY OF CONGRESS CATALOGING-IN-PUBLICATION DATA

Sheen, Barbara.
  Acne / by Barbara Sheen.
    v. cm. — (Diseases and disorders series)
Includes bibliographical references and index.
Contents: What is acne? — Diagnosis and treatment — Alternative and complementary
treatments — Living with acne — What the future holds.
  ISBN 1-59018-345-2 (hardback : alk. paper)
    1. Acne—Juvenile literature. 2. Skin—Diseases—Juvenile literature. [1. Acne. 2. Skin—
Care and hygiene.] I. Title. II. Series.
  RL131.S53 2004
  616.5'3—dc22
                                2003017747

Table of Contents

"The Most Difficult Puzzles Ever Devised"

CHARLES BEST, ONE of the pioneers in the search for a cure for diabetes, once explained what it is about medical research that intrigued him so. "It's not just the gratification of knowing one is helping people," he confided, "although that probably is a more heroic and selfless motivation. Those feelings may enter in, but truly, what I find best is the feeling of going toe to toe with nature, of trying to solve the most difficult puzzles ever devised. The answers are there somewhere, those keys that will solve the puzzle and make the patient well. But how will those keys be found?"

Since the dawn of civilization, nothing has so puzzled people—and often frightened them, as well—as the onset of illness in a body or mind that had seemed healthy before. A seizure, the inability of a heart to pump, the sudden deterioration of muscle tone in a small child—being unable to reverse such conditions or even to understand why they occur was unspeakably frustrating to healers. Even before there were names for such conditions, even before they were understood at all, each was a reminder of how complex the human body was, and how vulnerable.

While our grappling with understanding diseases has been frustrating at times, it has also provided some of humankind's most heroic accomplishments. Alexander Fleming's accidental discovery in 1928 of a mold that could be turned into penicillin has resulted in the saving of untold millions of lives. The isolation of the enzyme insulin has reversed what was once a death sentence for anyone with diabetes. There have been great strides in combating conditions for which there is not yet a cure, too. Medicines can help AIDS patients live longer, diagnostic tools such as mammography and ultrasounds can help doctors find tumors while they are treatable, and laser surgery techniques have made the most intricate, minute operations routine.

This "toe-to-toe" competition with diseases and disorders is even more remarkable when seen in a historical continuum. An astonishing amount of progress has been made in a very short time. Just two hundred years ago, the existence of germs as a cause of some diseases was unknown. In fact, it was less than 150 years ago that a British surgeon named Joseph Lister had difficulty persuading his fellow doctors that washing their hands before delivering a baby might increase the chances of a healthy delivery (especially if they had just attended to a diseased patient)!

Each book in Lucent's Diseases and Disorders series explores a disease or disorder and the knowledge that has been accumulated (or discarded) by doctors through the years. Each book also examines the tools used for pinpointing a diagnosis, as well as the various means that are used to treat or cure a disease. Finally, new ideas are presented—techniques or medicines that may be on the horizon.

Frustration and disappointment are still part of medicine, for not every disease or condition can be cured or prevented. But the limitations of knowledge are being pushed outward constantly; the "most difficult puzzles ever devised" are finding challengers every day.

A Disease That Is Often Ignored

F RED WAS TWELVE years old when he developed acne. At first he noticed white bumps under his skin. Then, small pimples with black tops appeared. Larger red pimples, many of which were filled with pus, followed. He explains:

> From the time I was twelve to eighteen was pretty miserable skin-wise. I had pimples on my face, neck, back, and upper arms. It was continuous; when one went away another one took its place. I'd go to school in the morning; in the afternoon I'd look in the mirror and I'd have a bunch of great big welts on my face that sprouted up while I was at school.

> It was humiliating. I used all my money on creams and med-icated pads. But they didn't help. My acne was too bad. I asked my parents to take me to a doctor for medicine. But my parents thought that seeing a doctor wouldn't help. They thought that acne was a part of growing up. They told me that it wasn't any-thing to take seriously. Everyone got acne and eventually it would go away with no harm done. In the meantime, I just had to live with it.[1]

Like many people, Fred's parents were misinformed about acne. Acne is not harmless. It is a disease that causes the development of pimples and cysts on the skin of millions of people, the major-ity of whom are teenagers. If acne is left untreated, it can lead to the development of permanent scars. Unfortunately, since acne is such a common condition, is not life threatening, and often dis-appears as a person ages, many people do not take acne seriously.

New York City dermatologist Dr. Bruce Katz explains: "Parents just don't get it. . . . Acne is not a trivial cosmetic problem to be waited out until pimples disappear on their own, but a medical condition that, left untreated, can leave youngsters with unsightly scars. . . . Acne should be taken very seriously."[2]

Although commonly perceived as a cosmetic problem, acne is actually a disease that causes emotional trauma and lasting physical damage like these scars.

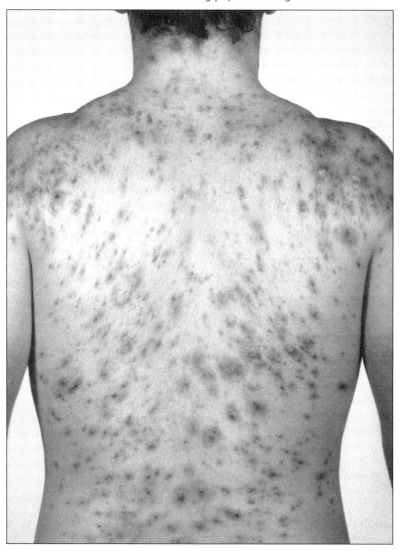

Making matters worse, because the seriousness of acne is often trivialized, many people with acne find themselves ridiculed or shunned by their peers. Instead of being treated with understanding, they are frequently teased or laughed at. Fred explains: "I took a lot of teasing. Any kid with acne was a target. Pizza Face, Hamburger Man, and Frankenstein were just a few of the names I was called."[3]

Even when people have no intention of being rude or hurtful, it is not uncommon for people with acne to be confronted by unpleasant reactions from strangers because acne visibly affects a person's appearance. A young man describes his experience:

> Me and some friends, there were about five of us, we were going to a birthday party at the house of one of my closest friend's cousins. I had never met the cousin before. . . . When we arrived, a pretty young woman opened the door and my friend started to introduce all of us. She greeted everyone with a warm smile and a kiss on the cheek, but when it was my turn to be introduced she just smiled politely and shook my hand. I felt that I repulsed her.[4]

Common Misconceptions

Ignorance about acne has led many people to believe common misconceptions—for example, that a lack of cleanliness or eating sweets can cause acne. These misconceptions make many people with acne wrongly feel that they are somehow responsible for their condition. Misperceptions may also cause other people to treat people with acne unsympathetically. An acne patient explains how her father's belief in one such misconception affected her:

> It was almost as if I had an enemy in the home as well as the enemy of acne, because it was his ignorance of acne and his ignorance of my feelings, which was belittling. If he saw me eating chocolate I'd be given "that look." You know . . . "you shouldn't be eating and enjoying that" . . . which, I think is fair to say, is a common reaction from family and friends.[5]

In order to counteract these and other misconceptions as well as improve the way individuals with acne are treated by others, it is important that everyone learn more about acne. By under-standing what causes acne, how it is treated, and how different be-haviors affect the disease, people with acne will be better able to cope. At the same time, learning about acne will help friends and family members to provide more support for their loved ones. Learning about acne will also help others become more sensitive about the way they interact with people with acne.

Indeed, once Fred and his family learned more about acne, his parents took him to the doctor, where he was given medicine that helped get his acne under control. Today, Fred is a grown man with his own family. In the years that have passed he has learned quite a bit about acne, and so have his parents. "When the grandkids started breaking out, my parents insisted they be taken to the doc-tor right away," Fred explains. "It took some time, but we've all learned just how serious acne is."[6]

Chapter 1

What Is Acne?

ACNE IS A COMMON skin disease that affects tiny ducts in the skin where hair grows. These ducts are known as follicles. Acne occurs when the follicles become clogged and infected. This causes sores known as acne lesions, or pimples, to develop on and under the skin.

Excess Hormones Cause Excess Oil Production

There are a number of factors that cause the follicles to become clogged and infected. One important factor is the overproduction of androgen. Androgen is a chemical, or male sex hormone, that both males and females normally produce. However, hormonal changes in the body during puberty, pregnancy, or the female menstrual cycle cause some people to produce higher than usual levels of androgen. Although scientists are unsure why, excess androgen stimulates the sebaceous oil glands inside the follicles to enlarge and manufacture excess amounts of oil called sebum. Whereas the normal production of sebum is necessary for healthy skin, excess sebum leads to the development of acne.

Normally, the sebaceous oil glands produce small amounts of sebum, whose job it is to moisten and protect the skin. In order to do this, sebum works its way up through the hair follicles, where it washes away dead cells that accumulate in the follicles. Then sebum empties onto the skin through tiny openings in the follicles called pores. Here sebum protects the skin from bacteria that live on the skin by washing the bacteria away.

However, when excess sebum is produced, it accumulates in the follicles rather than spilling out onto the surface of the skin. This occurs because the follicles are extremely small and narrow. Therefore, large volumes of sebum cannot pass through the follicles to the surface of the skin at the rate the sebum is produced. Instead, sebum becomes trapped in the follicles, where it mixes with dead skin cells, forms sticky plugs that block the pores, and prevents sebum from reaching the surface of the skin. As a result, the skin around the clogged follicles dries out. At the same time, since not every follicle becomes clogged, excess oil that spills onto the skin through unclogged follicles causes the skin to feel oily.

Clogged and infected hair follicles like this can cause sores, or acne lesions, to form under the skin.

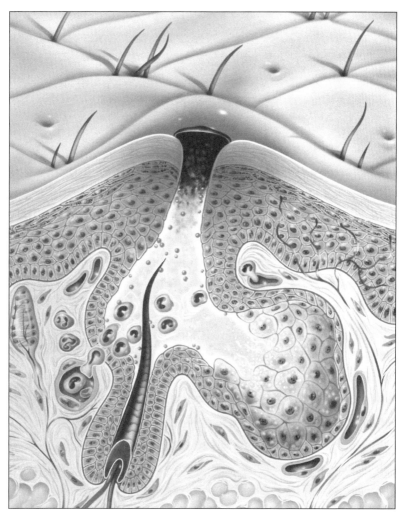

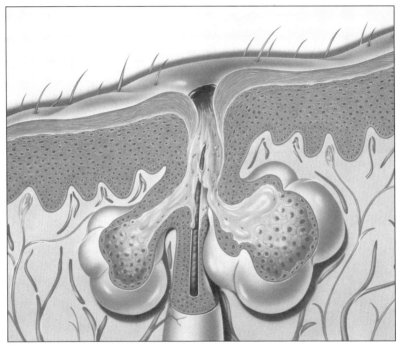

Infection occurs when bacteria enter a clogged hair follicle, causing the area around the follicle to become swollen and painful.

Therefore, a person with acne may have dry skin around clogged follicles and oily skin everywhere else.

Worse yet, without sebum to wash away bacteria on the skin, bacteria grow and multiply around the clogged follicles. Eventually, bacteria get inside the clogged follicles, where they mix with sebum and dead cells and cause an infection. This most commonly occurs on the parts of the body that have the largest sebaceous glands, such as the face, chest, neck, shoulders, upper back, and buttocks. The result is the development of one type of acne lesion known as a comedone.

Inflammation Makes Acne Worse

Unfortunately, the damage does not end there. Once bacteria enter the follicles, the immune system, which protects the body from infection and disease, reacts. Blood, rich with infection-fighting white blood cells, rushes to the area. As the infection worsens, pus and other powerful chemicals are also produced to combat the infection. This causes the infected area to become hot, red, swollen, and painful.

Heat, redness, swelling, pain, and the presence of pus are all characteristics of inflammation, which in the case of acne appears on the skin in the form of papules, pustules, and cysts, other types of acne lesions.

Different Types of Lesions

Whether a person develops comedones, papules, pustules, cysts, or a combination of these lesions depends on how severely the hair follicles are clogged and inflamed. The worse the inflammation, the more severe the acne lesion. For example, comedones, which are basically enlarged, clogged hair follicles, form before the hair follicles become inflamed or in the earliest stages of inflammation. Comedones contain sebum, dead skin cells, and bacteria that are trapped in the follicles, but comedones do not contain pus, nor are they red or swollen. That is why comedones are the least severe type of acne lesion.

Since comedones do not contain pus, they are quite small. All comedones have either a white or black tip. Hence, comedones are commonly known as whiteheads or blackheads.

Whiteheads and Blackheads

Whiteheads look like small white bumps and are usually about the size of a pinhead. They form under the skin as the follicles become more and more clogged and enlarged. Whiteheads never reach the skin's surface or open up. Therefore, they are called closed comedones.

Blackheads, on the other hand, are closed comedones that continue to grow upward until they break through the skin's surface. At this point, the enlarged hair follicle is visible and open to the skin's surface. For this reason, blackheads are known as open comedones.

To the naked eye the contents of an open comedone look black. The black color is the result of oxidation, a process of discoloration that occurs when dead cells, sebum, and bacteria mix with oxygen in the air. However, some people mistakenly think that dirt trapped under the skin causes an open comedone to appear black. A young man recalls how this misconception affected him: "I had blackheads all over my forehead and nose. I scrubbed my face constantly, trying to scrub the dirt out of those blackheads. But I kept getting more. I couldn't understand where all the dirt was coming from."[7]

Since comedones do not form as a result of severe inflammation, they are not painful, no matter whether they are blackheads or whiteheads. Moreover, because comedones are not large, red, or pus filled, when seen from a distance, the skin of people with comedones, especially those with whiteheads, appears relatively clear. However, because comedones are enlarged, clogged follicles, they do not disappear until the follicles unclog. This may not occur under normal circumstances until sebum production decreases or the patient receives effective acne treatment. Therefore, whiteheads and blackheads often stay on or under the skin for a long time.

Even more troubling, some closed comedones do not grow upward and become open comedones. Instead, as they become more and more packed with sebum, they grow downward under the surface of the skin and continue to enlarge until they burst. This results in the formation of more serious acne lesions such as papules and pustules.

Papules and Pustules

When closed comedones burst, their contents get into surrounding tissues. In response, the immune system sends more blood to the area, which causes inflammation to begin or worsen. As a result, the closed comedone and the area surrounding it become red and swollen. This redness and swelling appears on the skin in the form of a papule.

Papules are small, firm, red bumps. They are only mildly inflamed because they form before pus has reached the area. Therefore, papules are more severe acne lesions than comedones, but milder than acne lesions that contain pus. However, because papules are inflamed, they are often tender to the touch.

As the inflammation worsens, the immune system sends pus to the area. When this happens, pustules form. Because pustules are caused by severe inflammation, they often feel hot and may be quite sensitive to the touch.

Not surprisingly, pustules are larger than papules. They are often about the size of the tip of a person's little finger. Pustules are red at the base, with a yellowish, pus-filled inner region. A man who had pustules on his face, shoulders, and neck recalls: "They were big old welts filled with white poison and surrounded by red rings."[8]

Although a pustule's red base forms on the surface of the skin, the pus-filled core is near, but still underneath, the skin. However, as inflammation worsens and more pus is formed in the area, the pus-filled core of a pustule begins to swell like a balloon. When this happens, it is not uncommon for pustules to pop open and spill pus onto the skin. A man recalls: "In the morning before I went to school, I'd have big welts on my shoulders and neck. Sometimes at school they would break without me even knowing. When I got home I'd have stains on my shirt."[9]

Cysts

Just as worsening inflammation causes a pustule to expand upward through the skin's surface, worsening inflammation also causes pustules to expand downward. When this occurs, a cyst is

Papules like this are small, red bumps that form when a closed comedone bursts and spreads infection to surrounding tissue.

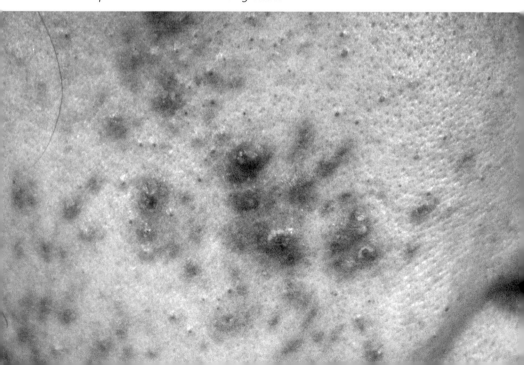

formed. Cysts are packed with large amounts of pus that extend deep below the skin's surface. Due to swelling, cysts may be several centimeters in diameter. Most cysts are red or purple and extremely painful. Since cysts form when inflammation and infection are the most severe, cysts are the most serious type of acne lesions.

Three Types of Acne

Just as there are different types of acne lesions, there are also different types of acne. Although there are a number of rare forms of acne, most experts divide acne into three main types: comedonal acne, acne vulgaris, and cystic acne.

The first type, comedonal acne, consists of whiteheads and blackheads alone, without the presence of other acne lesions. Therefore, comedonal acne is the mildest form of acne. However, since closed comedones often burst and become inflamed, it is not uncommon for people with comedonal acne eventually to develop papules and pustules.

When people have a mix of comedones, papules, and pustules, they have acne vulgaris, or common acne. A man who suffered from acne vulgaris recalls: "I had them all. I had blackheads on my nose. I had whiteheads on my forehead. I had bumpy red pimples and big pus pimples on my chin, neck, back, and shoulders."[10]

Acne vulgaris is the most common form of acne, affecting approximately 90 percent of all people with acne. Acne vulgaris can be mild, moderate, or severe, depending on the number of acne lesions a person has and how severely the lesions are inflamed.

The third type of acne, cystic acne, is the most severe form of acne. The presence of comedones, papules, pustules, and numerous acne cysts characterize cystic acne. Because cysts are caused by severe inflammation and infection, cystic acne can be quite painful.

Making matters worse, if cystic acne is left untreated, the severe inflammation and infection that cause cystic acne can damage surrounding tissues. This frequently leaves the skin of people with cystic acne permanently scarred. A patient explains: "You can see the scars where I had cysts today. They look like little craters. You can see them on my neck and on my back. I've got a little bit of evidence on my face too. Wherever you see a crater, that's where I had a cyst."[11]

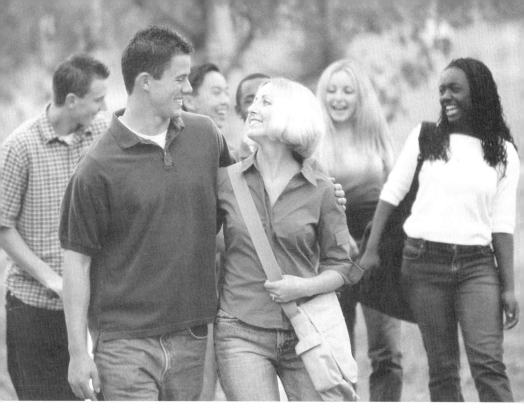

Although people of any age can develop acne, teenagers are most commonly affected by the disease.

People at Risk

Although almost everyone has an occasional whitehead or black-head, certain groups are more likely to develop acne vulgaris and cystic acne than others. These include adolescents, adult women, people under stress, people taking certain medications, and people whose parents had acne.

Acne in Adolescents

Adolescents are the largest group at risk of developing acne. This is because acne usually begins during puberty, when the body starts producing androgen. Androgen production is usually at its peak when people are between the ages of twelve and seventeen. Therefore, more oil is produced in the hair follicles of adolescents than in any other age group. As a result, experts estimate that more than 85 percent of all adolescents between the ages of twelve and seventeen develop some form of acne. This translates to more than 20 million teenagers in the United States. Moreover, although both males and females produce androgen, adolescent males produce ten times more androgen than females do because androgen is a male sex hormone. Consequently, it is not surprising that adolescent boys are more likely to develop severe cases of acne vulgaris as well as cystic acne; whereas teenage girls are more likely to develop comedonal acne and mild cases of acne vulgaris.

Generally, oil production decreases after the age of seventeen. In most cases, as androgen and sebum levels decrease, so does acne. Thus, by the time most adolescents reach age eighteen, their acne symptoms begin to subside and disappear. However, approximately 30 percent of all adolescents with acne continue to be plagued with acne for the rest of their lives. According to acne expert and dermatologist Anthony C. Chu, "Acne can persist well into old age and I have a number of patients in their sixties, seventies, and even eighties who still have active acne. Acne is, therefore, not merely a teenage occurrence; it can affect you at any time of your life." [12]

Adult Women and Acne

One group that is affected by acne well beyond adolescence is adult women. An estimated 5 percent of adult women have persistent acne that does not subside after puberty. An even larger number develop acne when they reach their twenties or thirties. Many of these women did not have acne as teenagers, while others had acne during their teen years that disappeared when puberty ended. Then, when these women reach their twenties or thirties, acne symptoms reappear as a result of fluctuating hormone levels caused by pregnancy, their monthly menstrual cycle, or hormonal imbalances. In fact, experts estimate that as many as 50 percent of all adult women suffer from acne. A woman describes her experience: "I had acne in high school. Luckily, it cleared up my senior year and my face was pretty clear through college. Now I am twenty-six, and started getting acne again." [13]

Some women experience only occasional acne flare-ups. Since the female menstrual cycle causes hormone levels to rise and fall, many experts believe these flare-ups occur when lower than normal levels of the female sex hormone, estrogen, are being produced. Estrogen is known to counterbalance the production of androgen. Therefore, without sufficient estrogen, androgen production increases unchecked, leading to acne flare-ups. At other times, when estrogen levels are high and androgen levels are low, these women's skin remains clear. Experts are unsure why this problem does not affect all women, but they theorize it is more likely to occur in women who, for unknown reasons, have the greatest fluctuation in their hormone levels.

Similarly, acne often flares up at different times during pregnancy as a pregnant woman's hormone levels change in order to accommodate her body's changing needs. Comparable hormonal changes often occur in some women after they give birth. As a result, some adult women develop acne shortly after their babies are born.

People Under Stress

Stress is another factor that can change hormone levels in adult women, men, and adolescents. Although scientists do not believe

People under stress, like this anxious bride, are at high risk of experiencing acne flare-ups.

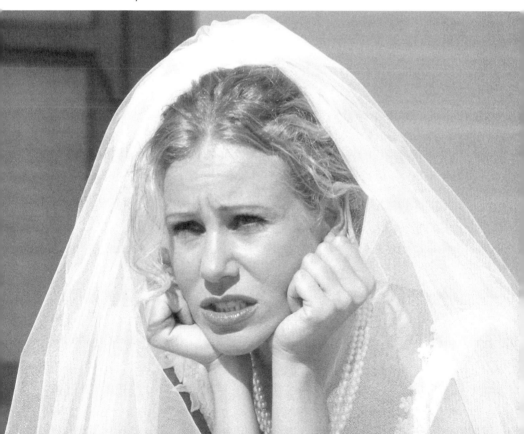

that stress directly causes acne, numerous studies have linked stress and acne flare-ups. The reason for this link is that when the body is under stress, it responds by producing hormones, including androgen and cortisol. Cortisol, like androgen, stimulates oil production. Therefore, people who are under stress are at risk of developing acne or having their existing acne worsen. Moreover, even though the production of stress hormones decreases as a person relaxes, stress-induced acne flare-ups often do not clear up until the inflammation heals. This may take a week or more.

Chu describes how stress affects his patients: "I have looked after four women who have cancelled their weddings on at least one occasion. Each time they neared their wedding day, stress levels increased and their spots became so bad that they cancelled because they could not bear the thought of wedding photographs of themselves covered with spots."[14]

People Taking Medication

Just as stress can change hormone levels, certain medications can also have this effect. For example, although some birth control pills contain estrogen, which lowers androgen levels, one type of birth

Keloid scars like this form when the skin produces too much collagen in an effort to heal an acne breakout.

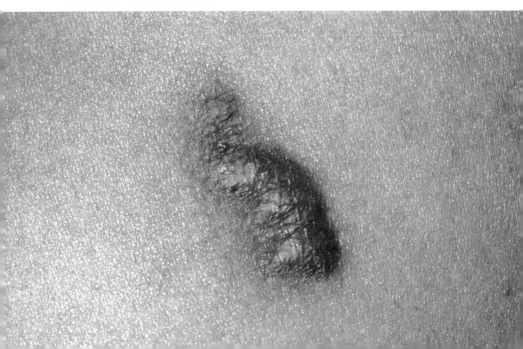

control pill contains progesterone, a hormone that stimulates the body to produce androgen, which can make acne worse. Other medicines such as those used to treat epilepsy, a disorder that causes seizures, and anabolic steroids, drugs often used illegally by athletes and bodybuilders to stimulate muscle growth, stimulate the production of androgen and have been linked to acne.

Genetics

Genetics also plays a role in determining who is at risk of developing acne. Experts agree that acne seems to run in families and that there seems to be a direct link between the development of severe acne and familial patterns. Experts are unsure why this is so, since an acne gene has not yet been discovered. However, a number of studies have shown that genetics does play a role in determining how likely a person is to develop acne. Various studies of identical twins, for example, found in over 50 percent of all cases that if one twin develops acne so does the other. Correspondingly, other studies have shown similarities among parents and children regarding the types of acne lesions, the severity of acne, and the duration of acne. A patient with acne explains: "I inherited it [acne] from my mother, and she's always telling me that she had the exact same thing and that it will go away. I am mad that I inherited it from her."[15]

Physical Effects of Acne

No matter who gets acne, acne can have a long-lasting physical effect. Acne lesions can leave permanent scars on an acne patient's skin. When a clogged hair follicle becomes infected, and the body sends white blood cells and powerful chemicals to combat the infection, swelling causes tissue around the infected follicle to be damaged. In many cases, once the infection is gone, the tissue is too damaged to return to its normal state. This damage appears in two distinct types of acne scars, scars caused by increased tissue formation and scars caused by tissue loss.

Scars caused by increased tissue formation are called keloid scars. Keloid scars form when the skin responds to tissue injury by producing an excess of collagen, a substance that helps the skin regenerate. Too much collagen causes the production of excess tissue to form over the damaged area. The results are keloid scars, which look like firm, shiny, flesh-colored lumps.

Acne scars that are caused by tissue loss occur when the body is unable to completely rebuild damaged tissue. Often called depressed, ice-pick, or pitted scars, these scars look like the skin has been pushed in, forming a soft depression with puckered edges. Pitted scars can be quite small, or they can be over a centimeter in diameter. Pitted scars are the most common type of acne scar and are commonly found on the face, back, and shoulders.

Fortunately, not every person who has acne develops acne scars. Doctors are unable to predict accurately whether or not a person with acne will develop scars. However, in most cases, as the severity of a person's acne increases so does the amount of tissue damage. Since acne scars result from damaged tissue, individuals who suffer the most tissue damage are most at risk of developing acne scars. Generally, these are individuals with severe cases of acne.

Emotional Effects of Acne

Even when acne does not cause permanent scars, because acne affects a person's appearance it can take an emotional toll on a person. People with acne often feel self-conscious about their appearance. Over time, their self-esteem and self-confidence decrease. This makes them feel insecure and anxious in social situations. In fact, many people with acne avoid social situations due to self-consciousness about their appearance. Indeed, many become shy and withdrawn. A young man explains: "I've lived with really heavy acne for the last five years. I feel so self-conscious that I don't even like going out. It's ruined my confidence." [16]

The combination of low self-esteem, embarrassment, and increasing social isolation leads many people with acne to become depressed. When people are depressed, they often lose interest in daily activities and feel tired, anxious, and unhappy. Some may contemplate suicide. In fact, according to a 2002 survey by the Acne Support Group, a British organization that helps acne sufferers, 15 percent of the acne patients surveyed reported feeling suicidal, and 75 percent reported feeling depressed because of acne. An acne patient describes how acne-caused depression affected her: "I did not look in mirrors whatsoever. I walked into a room and immediately shut out the light. Everything I did, I did in darkness because any time I caught a glimpse of myself I felt suicidal."[17]

Truly, many people with acne bear both emotional and physical scars all their lives. A former acne patient explains:

> It's easy to see the scars on my back and neck. What you can't see is what it did to me inside. I went from a fairly self-confident kid to an angry, withdrawn, and embarrassed teenager. Even today, the memories of the teasing and the embarrassment are quite vivid. It makes me queasy just to think about it. Even when the pimples are gone, acne stays with you a long time.[18]

Chapter 2

Diagnosis and Treatment

A CNE IS EASY TO diagnose. It is the only skin disease in which comedones are present. Other skin diseases, such as rosacea and skin rashes caused by allergies or insect bites, may have red lesions that resemble papules, but there is an absence of comedones. Therefore, the presence of comedones, whether alone or in combination with other skin lesions, indicates the presence of acne.

Treatment to Fit the Type and Severity of Acne

Once acne is diagnosed, the doctor evaluates the type and severity of a patient's lesions in order to determine what treatment is best. Acne treatment is individualized. It depends on the type of acne a person has as well as how severely acne lesions are inflamed. For example, treatment for whiteheads and blackheads focuses on removing dead skin cells that clog the follicles, while treatment for pustules is aimed at destroying infection and reducing inflammation. In an effort to achieve these different goals, different medications are needed.

The Acne Scale

To ensure that each patient receives the most effective treatment for his or her individual problems, doctors employ a special scale known as the acne grading scale. The acne grading scale rates the severity of acne on a scale from zero to eight, with zero indicating very mild acne and eight indicating very severe acne. For example, if a patient has a few comedones, he or she is given a zero rating. The rating increases with the number, size, and severity of a person's lesions. Therefore, a patient with half of his or her face

24

covered with papules, comedones, and a few pustules receives a four rating, which denotes moderate acne. A rating of eight indicates very severe acne, with the patient having acne lesions of all types, including numerous cysts, covering almost all of his or her face. Once a person's acne has been rated, doctors match the rating to specific treatment plans recommended by the American Academy of Dermatology, an organization that studies skin

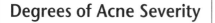

Degrees of Acne Severity

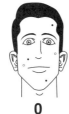

0
Few scattered comedones
(blackheads and whiteheads).

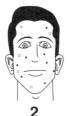

2
Thirty to forty papules and comedones
over one-fourth of the face.

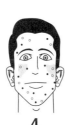

4
About half of the face has papules,
comedones, and a few pustules.
Some lesions are red and inflamed.

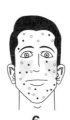

6
About three-fourths of the face is involved.
Many comedones, pustules,
some quite large.

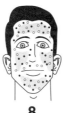

8
All or most of the face is involved.
Large, prominent pustules, much inflammation.
Healed lesions leave scars.

diseases. At the same time, the doctor makes adjustments in the recommended treatment for individual differences. For example, these differences may include such factors as how dry or oily the patient's skin may be, the patient's gender, whether the patient is allergic to any medications, and whether the patient is pregnant or planning to become pregnant soon.

A Common Goal

Because there are many differences in the severity and types of acne lesions, there are a wide variety of acne treatment options. These include over-the-counter medication people can purchase without a doctor's prescription as well as more powerful, doctor-prescribed medications. Acne medication may be taken orally or applied directly onto the skin in the form of a topical treatment. Often, oral and topical treatments are combined. Once acne outbreaks are eliminated, a special type of surgery known as skin dermabrasion can lessen acne scars.

No matter what form of treatment is used, all acne treatments share a common goal: to control the sequence of events that cause acne outbreaks in order to prevent new outbreaks from occurring. Experts agree that since there are so many different acne treatment options available, most cases of acne outbreaks can be controlled. Edmonton, Canada, dermatologist Don Groot explains: "We've got acne by the tail now. If we catch it early, you can do wonders with acne. It's not a difficult disease to treat anymore."[19]

Topical Treatments

Some of the most popular and effective treatment options available for acne are topical treatments. Most commonly used to treat cases of mild to moderate acne, topical treatments come in cream, lotion, or gel form and on specially prepared pads. Those used to treat the mildest cases of acne can be purchased without a doctor's prescription.

Salicylic Acid

Salicylic acid is a popular topical treatment that can be purchased without a doctor's prescription. Salicylic acid does not treat infection or inflammation. Therefore, it is mainly used to treat comedones.

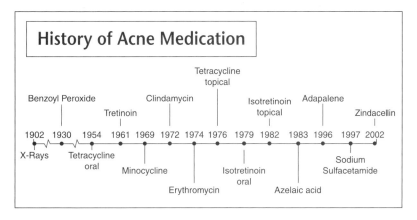

History of Acne Medication

When salicylic acid is rubbed onto the skin, it penetrates the pores and gets inside clogged hair follicles. Salicylic acid causes the dead skin cells inside the follicles to dissolve. This allows oil trapped in the follicles to reach the skin. Many patients report that treatment with salicylic acid helps eliminate acne outbreaks. A patient explains: "I have blackheads on my back. I wipe my back with salicylic acid wipes every night. It didn't help immediately, but after about a month, I noticed a difference. I think it's helping."[20]

Benzoyl Peroxide

Benzoyl peroxide is another topical treatment that can be purchased without a doctor's prescription. In fact, it is the main ingredient in most over-the-counter acne preparations. Used to treat mild inflammatory acne, benzoyl peroxide is available in different strengths. It is often used with products that contain salicylic acid by patients who have both comedones and mildly inflamed pustules.

Benzoyl peroxide is an oxidizing agent, meaning it releases oxygen. The bacteria that cause acne can only exist in an oxygen-free environment, such as a clogged hair follicle. When benzoyl peroxide penetrates hair follicles and releases oxygen, acne-causing bacteria are killed. This not only relieves existing infection but also stops new pustules from forming. A young woman describes her experience with benzoyl peroxide: "After two and a half weeks I was clearer than I had been since before puberty.... Using this benzoyl peroxide . . . has really changed the way I feel about myself and my ability to take on the world."[21]

Other Antibacterial Ointments and Vitamin A

In addition to benzoyl peroxide, there are a number of other antibacterial ointments used to treat mild inflammatory acne. These ointments contain chemicals such as sulfur that kill bacteria. In addition, there are a number of stronger antibiotic creams, gels, and lotions that contain powerful bacteria-killing drugs such as tetracycline and erythromycin, which are used to treat moderately inflamed acne. Although these products do control infection, they have no effect on clogged hair follicles. Therefore, these products are often combined with salicylic acid or a more powerful prescription-strength ointment such as Retin A, a popular retinoid.

In addition to topical treatments, doctors prescribe a variety of oral medications to treat acne.

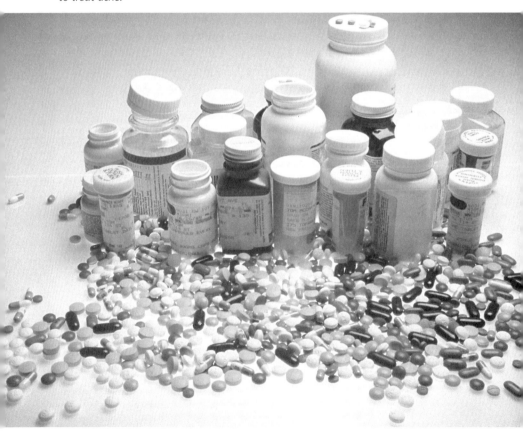

Retinoids are derived from vitamin A, which has a potent effect on the skin. Scientists have found that when vitamin A is applied to the skin, it slows the growth of skin cells. This is important in preventing acne because when new skin cells form, old skin cells are shed. Slowing the growth of skin cells keeps dead skin cells from building up inside the hair follicles. This stops new comedones from forming. In addition, for reasons that scientists cannot explain, vitamin A slows down oil production and stimulates the production of collagen. This gives the skin a smoother appearance. Therefore, vitamin A is often used to help smooth out acne scars. According to the American Academy of Dermatology: "Vitamin A products can make a big difference in the appearance of the skin. They speed [collagen] cell turnover and slow down oil production."[22]

Oral Medication

In addition to topical treatments, many people with moderate to severe inflammatory acne take oral medication, either alone or in combination with topical ointments. There are three main types of oral medications used to treat acne. They are antibiotics, hormones, and isotretinoin.

Antibiotics

Bacteria-fighting oral antibiotics such as tetracycline, erythromycin, clindamycin, and doxycycline are often prescribed for people whose acne does not respond to topical antibiotic treatment. Oral antibiotics are absorbed through the digestive system, into the bloodstream, and then into the skin and hair follicles. Here they kill acne-causing bacteria and reduce inflammation. This helps stop new acne lesions from forming and gives the skin a healthier appearance by lessening redness. However, most oral antibiotics are absorbed into the bloodstream quickly. Consequently, they are eliminated from the body rapidly. Therefore, in order to maintain a constant level of bacteria-fighting medication in the bloodstream, oral antibiotics must be taken frequently for an extended period of time. Indeed, some people with acne take antibiotics two or three times each day for six months to a year. Moreover, once treatment with oral antibiotics is stopped, unchecked bacteria often cause new acne outbreaks. In an effort to prevent this from occurring, when the skin begins to clear, treatment with oral antibiotics is gradually tapered off, rather than stopped abruptly, and replaced with topical antibiotic treatment. This helps restrain the growth of acne-causing bacteria.

Despite these drawbacks, treatment with oral antibiotics can be quite successful. A patient describes how treatment with tetracycline helped him. "I used benzoyl peroxide and medicated pads, but they didn't help. My acne was too bad. It took tetracycline to get it under control. It helped a lot, not 100 percent, but a lot. Even with the tetracycline, I still had some little pimples, but not those big old welts. Once the tetracycline kicked in I wasn't embarrassed about my appearance anymore."[23]

Hormones

For many teenage girls as well as women with adult-onset acne, treatment with female sex hormones such as estrogen offers another treatment option. Usually taken in the form of low-dose birth control pills, hormonal therapy increases the level of female hormones in a woman's bloodstream. This reduces or blocks the production of androgen. Once androgen production is decreased, sebum production is decreased as well. The result is decreased acne outbreaks. A woman describes her experience with hormone therapy: "I was surprised when my doctor prescribed birth control pills to clear up my skin. It sounded strange. But I was at the end of my rope as far as my skin was concerned. I tried just about everything else, so I decided to give birth control pills a shot. I am so happy with the results. My skin hasn't looked this good in years."[24]

Isotretinoin

For patients with severe cystic acne or for patients with moderate inflammatory acne that has proven to be resistant to oral antibiotics, isotretinoin is the most effective acne treatment available. In fact, it is the only medication that effectively controls severe cystic acne. Commonly sold under the brand name Accutane, isotretinoin is a vitamin A derivative that is administered in pill form.

Isotretinoin is an extremely powerful drug that stops all the changes in the skin that cause acne. It kills bacteria and reduces in-

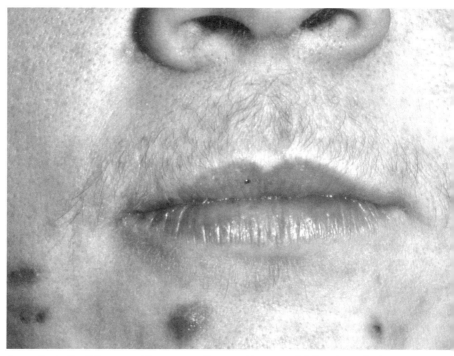

For patients like this man with severe cystic acne, the powerful drug isotretinoin has proven to be the most effective treatment available.

flammation. At the same time, it shrinks the sebaceous oil glands, reducing sebum production by up to 90 percent. It also slows up the growth of skin cells, which helps unblock hair follicles. Unclogging the hair follicles allows pustules and cysts trapped below the surface of the skin to work their way to the surface of the skin, where they burst and heal. Consequently, many patients find that their acne actually worsens in the first month of Accutane treatment but starts improving thereafter. Anthony C. Chu explains: "In the first month on Roaccutane [the name for isotretinoin in Great Britain] acne can worsen. . . . In most patients acne slowly reduces in the first two months, but there is then a more rapid response and, again in most patients, the acne clears completely in four months."[25]

Taken for a period of four to nine months, isotretinoin is effective in 98 percent of all cases. However, in some cases acne symptoms return after isotretinoin treatment ends. In these cases, patients may begin a second cycle of isotretinoin treatment. A patient describes her experience:

> After a few weeks on Accutane, my breakouts stopped dead in their tracks. I experienced no breakouts whatsoever for the remainder of the time I took the prescription. People with fantastic skin would come up to me and say, "I wish I had your skin." It was pretty incredible. However . . . I was not one of the lucky ones. Although my skin has been more manageable since Accutane, I have experienced serious breakouts since ending my cycle. Even so, I remain very thankful that I took it. I would describe my acne now as light to moderate thanks to Accutane, and with my current regime [use of topical treatments] I stay clear.[26]

Treating Acne Scars

Although acne medication can lessen and even eliminate acne outbreaks, many patients are left with permanent scars. For these patients, treatment with a form of surgery known as skin dermabrasion can help give the skin a smoother appearance. In this procedure, patients are given a local anesthetic to eliminate pain. Then, a high-speed instrument that resembles a wire brush is used to scrape away the top layer of skin and alter the contour of acne scars. Small scars may be completely removed, while the depth of large scars is reduced considerably. Because the top layer of skin is removed, after the procedure the patient's skin often appears red and may remain red for a month or more. However, according to Chu, once the skin heals, 70 percent of people who undergo skin dermabrasion report improvement in the appearance of their skin.

Risks and Side Effects of Acne Treatments

Despite the benefits of acne treatments, like all surgery and medication, those used for acne can cause side effects and health risks. For example, as in all surgical procedures, people who undergo skin dermabrasion can develop an infection or have an allergic reaction to the anesthetic.

Acne medicines too, present health risks. Topical ointments, for instance, can dry out and irritate the skin, causing it to become red and scaly. Retin A, in particular, makes the skin extremely sensitive to sunlight. If it is left on the skin when an individual goes out in direct sunlight, he or she is likely to experience a severe sunburn.

Oral antibiotics can also present problems for some patients by causing nausea, dizziness, stomachaches, and sensitivity to the sun. Furthermore, because oral antibiotics kill bacteria, they alter the level of normal bacteria present throughout the body. In women, lack of normal bacteria can lead to the growth of yeast in the vagina. This often causes the development of a yeast infection.

Oral antibiotics used for acne treatment can cause side effects in some patients, including skin irritation, nausea, and muscular pain.

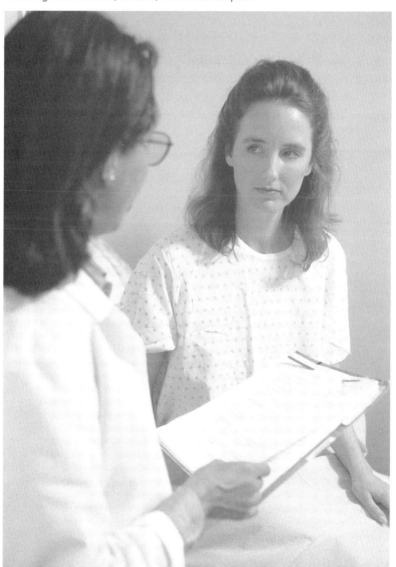

More troubling is the fact that long-term use of antibiotics can cause people to develop a resistance to these drugs. This can be devastating if a person develops a serious bacterial infection, such as bacterial pneumonia or strep throat, that requires antibiotics to be cured.

Hormones, too, can cause side effects such as mood swings, depression, and weight gain. An acne patient recalls: "I . . . took antibiotics so long that I have become very resistant to many of them. The doctors even tried birth control pills, the only real results from that was an extra twenty pounds!"[27] Hormone therapy has also recently been linked to an increased risk of breast cancer and heart disease.

Isotretinoin and Serious Health Problems

Even more disturbing are the health problems that isotretinoin can cause. Like Retin A, isotretinoin dries out the skin. However, because of its potency, its drying effect can cause the skin on the lips, fingers, toes, feet, and palms of the hands to swell, peel off, and bleed. Isotretinoin can also cause frequent nosebleeds, dry tear ducts, and muscular pain. In most cases, these problems disappear when treatment with isotretinoin ends, but in a few cases these problems persist indefinitely.

An article in the January 18, 2003, edition of the *Australian*, an Australian newspaper, describes one young man's experience:

> Ryan Burrows stood in the shower wearing pink dishwashing gloves to prevent his hands from bleeding, and all he could think was that his life had become "a living hell." For Burrows . . . the swollen hands, "which would bleed and ooze pus" if he shook anyone's hand or if they became wet were just one of the horrorific side effects he attributed to the acne treatment Roaccutane [the common name for isotretinoin in Australia]. . . . The dermatologist told Burrows any side effects would disappear as soon as he stopped taking the drug. Two-and-a-half years later, specialists cannot explain the shooting pains in his legs and feet. His lips still bleed unless he uses lip balm constantly.[28]

In addition, isotretinoin can permanently damage the liver, which filters drugs out of the body. Isotretinoin can also cause the texture of a person's hair to change temporarily and lead to temporary hair loss. A patient who was being treated with Accutane describes her experience: "Accutane produced the worst breakout I had ever experienced, along with scalp dryness. With hair down to the middle of my back, I was sure the talk of possible hair loss would happen to me. I quit."[29]

Isotretinoin and Psychiatric Problems

Isotretinoin has also been linked to psychiatric problems such as depression, violent behavior, and suicide attempts. Scientists do not know why a drug that targets the skin affects the brain. They theorize that isotretinoin may lower serotonin levels in the brain. Low levels of this brain chemical have been linked to depression, violence, and suicide. However, this link is controversial. It is unclear whether isotretinoin actually causes these problems or if the emotional impact of acne itself, combined with normal mood swings common to adolescents, is the cause. According to the Food and Drug Administration (FDA), a government agency that sets standards and regulations for the safe use of drugs, between 1982 and 2000, 147 people being treated with Accutane either committed suicide or were hospitalized for suicide attempts. The administration also reported one hundred violent acts committed by people taking Accutane in 2002. One such act involved an Accutane patient who flew a small airplane into a skyscraper in Tampa, Florida, in January 2002, damaging the building and killing himself.

The number of attempted and actual suicides among Accutane users, according to Hoffman-La Roche, the drug company that manufactures the drug, is comparatively lower than that for all U.S. citizens ages fifteen to twenty-four, the age group most likely to be treated with Accutane. But for individuals who experience psychiatric problems while taking isotretinoin and their families, the danger that the drug presents seems clearer. For instance, Accutane has been implicated in the 2002 suicide of a fourteen-year-old in Palo Alto, California, who jumped in front of a commuter train while being treated with the drug. It is also a possible factor in the 2000 suicide of Michigan congressman

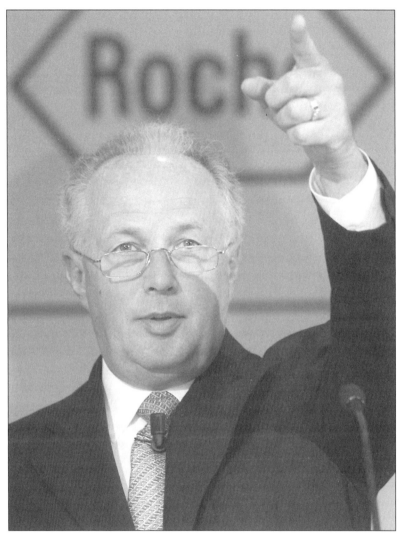

An executive for the drug company Hoffman-La Roche speaks about the psychological effects of Accutane, a drug linked to two patient suicides.

Bart Stupak's son. According to the congressman, "The side effects of Accutane are not worth it."[30] In fact, the congressman would like to see to the drug banned until further studies into its psychiatric effects are completed.

Although the drug has not been banned, due to these and other cases it is illegal for doctors to administer the drug until patients read a detailed medical guide, which describes the possible health risks that isotretinoin presents. The patient must then sign a consent form stating he or she is aware of the risks.

Isotretinoin and Birth Defects

Another health risk that female patients are warned about in the medical guide is the risk of damage to unborn babies. Because everything that enters an expectant mother's bloodstream also enters the fetus's bloodstream, when expectant mothers take isotretinoin, the drug's powerful effect can harm the developing fetus. According to the FDA, 35 percent of babies born to mothers treated with the drug during their pregnancies are born with birth defects. These defects include physical deformities, undeveloped organs, blindness, and mental retardation. Isotretinoin can also cause the death of the fetus before birth, premature births, or the death of the newborn baby.

For this reason, the FDA prohibits the dispensation of isotretinoin to pregnant women. In addition, female patients must take two pregnancy tests before the drug can be prescribed, and women are warned not to become pregnant while taking the drug. Therefore, birth control is mandatory for sexually active women taking isotretinoin, as are monthly pregnancy tests. In addition, women are warned not to become pregnant for at least one month after stopping use of isotretinoin, since it takes at least one month for the drug to clear a person's system. A fifteen-year-old who took Accutane recalls her experience: "My doctor asked me if there's any chance I was pregnant—right in front of my mother. It was embarrassing to go for the pregnancy test every month."[31]

Despite the controversy surrounding isotretinoin and the side effects and possible health risks of other acne treatments, it is clear that acne treatments can lessen acne symptoms and help people have smoother, clearer skin. "Sure there were health risks," a former acne patient explains. "But I still can remember the teasing, embarrassment, and humiliation the pimples caused. That was a hundred times more dangerous and painful than anything any medicine could possibly do to me. Getting treatment changed my life."[32]

Chapter 3

Alternative and Complementary Treatments

S INCE ACNE MEDICATION can have harmful side effects, many people with acne explore alternative treatments in an effort to find safer treatment options. Moreover, some people with acne use alternative treatments to reduce stress, which, when left unchecked, encourages acne outbreaks. Indeed, the use of alternative treatments has grown widely among acne patients, with many reporting positive results. An acne patient explains why she sought alternative treatment:

> The doctor prescribed Retin A. It totally dried out my skin. It even hurt to smile. If anything my face was redder and more inflamed than when I started. I looked like a burn victim! Then, my cousin started using tea tree oil and her skin looked great. She swore by it. She said that it was soothing and gentler than bp [benzoyl peroxide] or Retin A. That's when I decided to switch. After that, one thing led to another. The tea tree oil was great, but I still wasn't totally clear. I started checking out other natural treatments. Now I'm using tea tree oil and zinc, and doing some meditation. My skin's not perfect, but it's a whole lot better, and I feel better about myself.[33]

What Are Alternative and Complementary Treatments?

An alternative treatment is a form of treatment that, because of limited studies into its effectiveness and safety, is not approved for use or regulated by the FDA. In fact, rather than exacting scientific tests that are used in studying conventional treatments, alternative treatments often use anecdotal evidence to prove their effectiveness. Such evidence, which is based on reports by patients on how the treatment worked for them, does not usually include a

Alternative treatments for acne include homeopathic medications like these that are not regulated by the FDA.

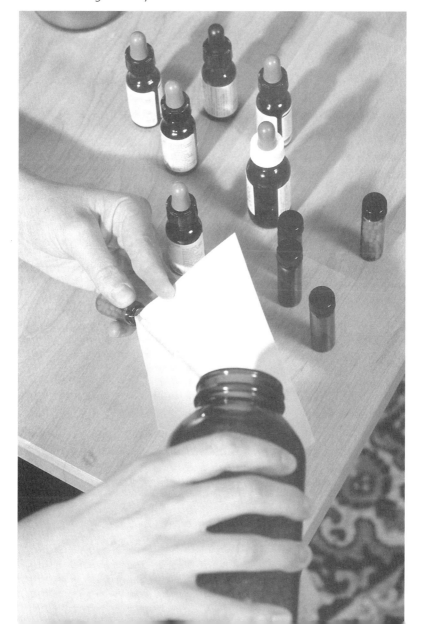

control group or report any negative results. Consequently, most alternative treatments are not widely prescribed by traditional health care providers in the United States, who depend on the government to verify that the advantages of conventional treatments surpass any likely health risks.

Despite these issues, many health care professionals believe that several alternative treatments are effective in treating acne, especially when they are combined with conventional acne treatments in a method known as complementary treatment. Doctors recommend complementary treatment because it can regulate hormones, reduce inflammation, fight infection, and reduce stress.

Three Types of Alternative Treatments for Acne

The most widely used alternative treatments for acne fall into three categories—those that are taken internally, those that are applied on the skin, and those that eliminate stress. Dietary supplements such as herbs, vitamins, and minerals are among the most popular internal treatments. In fact, herbal remedies have been used to treat many diseases, including acne, for thousands of years, and herbs still remain the primary treatment for acne in China and Thailand.

Herbal remedies use the leaves, roots, and stems of plants that are known to have healing properties. Usually taken ground up in capsule form or as a tea, herbal remedies for acne consist of herbs that balance hormone levels, boost the immune system, and reduce inflammation. Because herbs are natural, many people feel that they are gentler and safer than conventional medicines.

Herbs That Balance Hormone Levels

Herbs that balance hormone levels are the most commonly prescribed herbs for acne. They include chaste berry, red clover, black cohosh, wild yam, evening primrose, and dong quai, all of which are prescribed for women. These herbs contain phytoestrogen, a plant-based female hormone-like compound. Therefore, although they are useful for women, they are inappropriate for males due to chemical differences in the male and female body.

Herbalists believe phytoestrol increases the effect of the female sex hormone, estrogen, on the body while counterbalancing the ef-

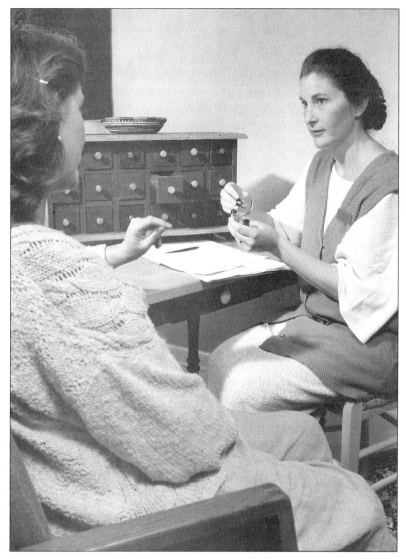

An acne patient consults with an herbalist about herbal treatments. Herbs most commonly prescribed for acne act to balance the patient's hormone levels.

fect of androgen. Although studies into the effectiveness of hormone-balancing herbs on acne are limited, many experts think herbs containing phytoestrogen can help women with hormonal acne. Stanley W. Beyrle, a naturopathic doctor at the Kansas Clinic of Traditional Medicine in Wichita, explains:

Black cohosh works as a regulator or a normalizer of the female reproductive system [the part of a woman's body that produces female sex hormones] by helping to restore hormone balance. When it comes to gynecological complaints [conditions such as hormonal acne that involve female sex hormones and sex organs], there isn't a better herb than black cohosh.[34]

Herbs to Combat Infection and Inflammation

Other herbs used to treat acne, such as echinacea, burdock, licorice, and dandelion root, are thought to contain compounds that attack bacteria, thus reducing infection and inflammation. Herbs like salvia and red peony, on the other hand, are thought to improve circulation and tissue growth, which increases the skin's ability to heal. The effect of these herbs on acne patients has been studied in China. There they are commonly prescribed for acne in individually formulated combinations based on each patient's particular skin problems. Such combinations are also prescribed for acne patients by practioners of Chinese herbal medicine in the United States and other Western countries. An acne patient who was treated with such an herbal combination explains: "It did work. It's all rather mysterious, with all the herbs, and it's a slow and gradual effect, but it [the patient's acne] calmed down and six months later it's still under control."[35]

Vitamins and Minerals

Treatment with vitamins and minerals, in particular vitamin B_5, is another widely used alternative treatment for acne. Also known as pantothenic acid, vitamin B_5 is believed by some experts to be as effective in reducing the production of sebum as isotretinoin.

Treatment with vitamin B_5 is based on a theory developed by acne expert Dr. Lit-Hung Leung in 1995 in Hong Kong that a deficiency of vitamin B_5 leads to the development of acne. According to Leung, the body needs vitamin B_5 in order to process fat. When there is a shortage of vitamin B_5, fat that is normally burned for fuel or stored in cells for future use cannot be processed properly. Instead, it accumulates in the bloodstream. Since excess fat in the bloodstream can damage the body by clogging arteries and veins, the body tries to eliminate it. One way the body does this is by producing excess sebum, to which fat binds. In this way, excess fat in the form of sebum is eliminated through the skin. Thus, according to Leung's theory, the presence of excess fat in the bloodstream causes the body to increase sebum production in an effort to eliminate fat. This causes or worsens acne lesions. Therefore, when acne patients increase the level of vitamin B_5 in their bodies, they improve the processing of fat. This insures that fat is burned for energy or stored for future use instead of being used to produce excess sebum.

To test his theory, Leung sponsored a clinical trial in which he treated one hundred acne patients in Central Hospital in Hong Kong in 1997 with vitamin B_5. The patients, who had various severities of acne, were given ten grams of vitamin B_5 per day in capsule form. Although vitamin B_5 is present in many foods, including beans, nuts, oatmeal, and brewer's yeast, Leung says that some people with acne are so deficient in vitamin B_5 that they cannot get enough of it through food alone.

The study proved successful. Within six months, 90 percent of the subjects' acne had cleared. These results suggested to Leung that vitamin B_5 is an effective acne treatment. Many people concur with Leung. An acne patient who is currently using vitamin B_5 describes the results: "Though my skin isn't 100 percent clear yet, it's made excellent progress in that direction over the past five weeks. Far fewer breakouts overall and the oiliness of my skin has definitely decreased."[36]

Treatments That Are Applied to the Skin

Like herbs and vitamin B_5, topical alternative treatments usually consist of vitamins and minerals or natural ingredients derived from plants. One such popular alternative treatment is tea tree oil, which is applied directly onto pustules. Tea tree oil is an essential oil derived from the Australian ti tree. It is a natural antiseptic that destroys bacteria and draws out impurities, like pus, from acne lesions.

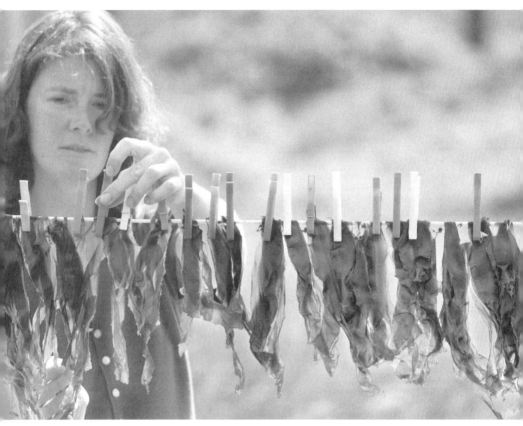

A biologist hangs seaweed to dry. Studies suggest that topical creams made with seaweed have a powerful effect on acne-causing bacteria.

Seaweed, too, has powerful antibacterial properties. First discovered in 2001 in France as a treatment for acne, topical treatments made from seaweed are quite potent. According to a November 2001 report in YM.com, the online edition of *YM* magazine, seaweed has such a powerful effect on acne-causing bacteria that it takes only two pounds of seaweed to make a ton of acne spot cream.

Other external herbal remedies use herbs such as agrimony, burdock, cloves, lavender, licorice root, and white willow, to name just a few, because of their anti-inflammatory, antiseptic, and pore-cleansing properties. In fact, white willow contains a natural form of salicylic acid. Often these herbs are combined with minerals such as zinc, which aid in the healing of skin tissue, and are applied on the skin systematically in the form of daily cleansers and healing balms and weekly facial masks. A woman whose grandson used such a system describes how it helped him: "My grandson was teased by the horrible acne covering his face. Now there is no sign he ever had acne. Within days of starting your system [one manufacturer's herbal skin care regime] his acne turned to small scabs and then healed without scars. It also worked wonders on his chest and back."[37]

Ear Acupuncture

Acupuncture is another alternative treatment that is applied to the skin. Developed thousands of years ago in China, acupuncture is based on the concept that everyone has an energy known as chi flowing through their bodies. When this energy flow is blocked, illness occurs. In order to unblock this energy flow, acupuncturists insert small needles into specific points on the body. Acupuncturists think that some of these points, especially those found in the ear, control energy flow to the face, where acne is likely to occur. Therefore, inserting needles into the ear stimulates the flow of energy to the face. Once the flow is restored, blood circulation to the face improves, bringing increased oxygen, collagen, nutrients, and infection-fighting chemicals to acne-affected areas. In addition, acupuncturists believe that acupuncture treatment balances hormone production.

Despite the lack of evidence proving that chi exists, a number of studies have shown acupuncture to be an effective treatment for acne. For example, one 1989 Chinese study reported in the *Journal of Traditional Chinese Medicine* treated eighty patients with moderate to severe acne with ear acupuncture every other day for a total of sixteen treatments. Seventy-seven percent of the patients were reported completely cured, while the skin of 14 percent showed a marked improvement. A 1990 Chinese study reported similar results.

Another study conducted at the University of Heidelberg, Germany, in 1992 investigated the effects of ear acupuncture on women with hormonal acne. In this study, half the subjects were treated with conventional hormone therapy, and half were treated with acupuncture. At the study's conclusion, researchers reported that the skin of subjects treated with acupuncture was more improved than that of subjects treated with hormones. In addition, unlike the subjects treated with hormones, the subjects treated with acupuncture experienced no side effects.

Based on these and other studies, many medical doctors support the use of acupuncture as an acne treatment. Dr. Palle Rosted, a medical doctor and acupuncturist at Weston Park Hospital in Sheffield, England, reports on the benefit of acupuncture as an acne treatment: "The various studies generally testify to many cases of total recovery, and for the remaining patients a considerable degree of improvement."[38]

Treatments That Relieve Stress

Whereas some patients use alternative treatments as a substitute for conventional medicines, other patients combine conventional treatments with stress-relieving alternative treatments. Since controlling stress reduces the release of the hormone cortisol, which stimulates sebum production, controlling stress reduces the severity of acne. The most popular stress-relieving treatments for acne include relaxation response therapy, yoga, and aromatherapy.

Relaxation response therapy involves using the mind to help lower stress and thus reduce acne outbreaks. There are a number of ways acne patients do this. One way is through the use of relaxation tapes. Just as the name implies, relaxation tapes are audiotapes specifically designed to help listeners relax. Such tapes help listeners to concentrate their minds on relaxation by guiding them through a serious of exercises. The exercises provide acne patients instructions on ways to slow their breathing and relax their muscles, which reduce the body's response to stress. At the same time, the tapes often offer soothing background sounds such as the sound of the ocean or a gentle rain, which help listeners clear their minds of distressful thoughts. Relaxation tapes have proven so useful that the Acne Support Group, the largest acne support group in Great Britain, has developed tapes specifically for its members.

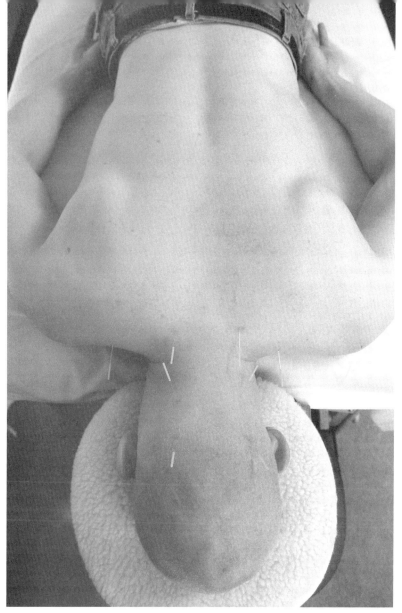

An effective method of acne treatment, acupuncture involves inserting fine needles into the skin to improve blood circulation in affected areas.

Meditation and Guided Imagery

While some people with acne use relaxation tapes to help con-centrate their minds on relaxation, others use meditation or guided imagery to achieve similar results. Meditation involves using con-centration techniques to clear the mind in order to relax the body and relieve stress. While meditating, people silently repeat a word or phrase until they feel calm and all stressful thoughts are removed from their minds. Research has shown that during meditation, the production of cortisol decreases and remains lowered when individuals practice meditation often. As a result, sebum production and acne outbreaks are reduced.

Guided imagery is a type of meditation in which people center their thoughts on relaxing and healing their bodies. For example, when faced with a stressful situation, many acne patients use guided imagery to imagine themselves in a tranquil environment, such as a forest or beach, where they feel relaxed and happy. At the same time, they envision their complexion without acne. The feelings evoked during guided imagery help people with acne lower their stress levels and strengthen their resolve to heal. An acne patient explains:

> I light scented candles, pop in a CD, and imagine myself walking on the beach in Mazatlan [a beach resort in Mexico]. I think about how good I feel, how peaceful the beach is, and how the sun warms my face and heals my skin. I imagine the sun cleansing and clearing my skin from the outside, and my own body doing it from the inside. In my mind, my skin is perfect and I'm beautiful. When I'm done, I'm relaxed and more confident, too. [39]

Yoga

Practicing yoga, a form of exercise that originated in ancient India, is another way people with acne relieve stress. Yoga exercises involve slow, controlled stretching and breathing, which relax the body while lowering cortisol levels. Because yoga is a form of exercise, it also improves blood circulation. Improved circulation brings more oxygen and bacteria-fighting cells to areas affected by acne. Yoga practitioners say that specific yoga postures such as the lion, standing and seated sun, and cobra have distinct healing effects on the body, including relaxation, internal cleansing, and releasing blocked energy. Although there is little proof that yoga does all these things, it is so popular for reducing stress that many physicians recommend it to their patients.

Many acne patients find yoga to be effective in reducing stress as well as improving their complexion. They report feeling more relaxed and calm, along with seeing a noticeable improvement in the brightness and healthiness of their skin.

Aromatherapy

Aromatherapy is another popular alternative treatment for reducing stress. It is based on the theory that scent influences the

By helping to alleviate stress, yoga can help improve the complexion of acne sufferers.

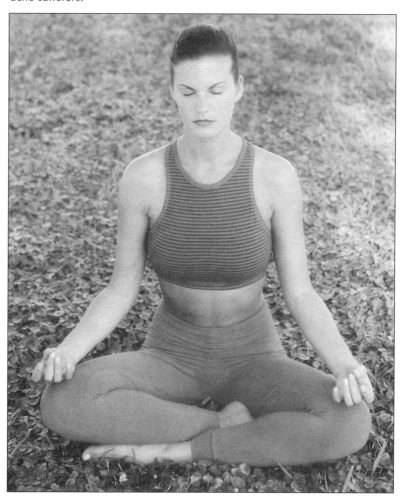

way people feel. Aromatherapy uses candles scented with essential oils extracted from plants. It also uses aroma lamps and diffusers that spray the oil into the air in a mist. These oils are derived from plants such as jasmine, chamomile, vanilla, lemon balm, and lavender and are believed to have calming properties. Indeed, people report feeling calmer and less stressed after inhaling them.

A man shops for herbal remedies. Although some people consider alternative treatments to be safer than conventional treatments, such therapies still pose health risks.

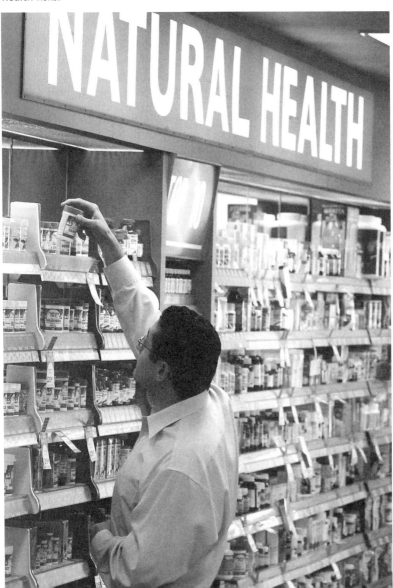

Studies into the effectiveness of aromatherapy are limited. However, neurologists at the Smell and Taste Treatment and Research Foundation in Chicago have been conducting research on aromatherapy for seventeen years. Their findings support the theory that scent has a powerful effect on an individual's mood and behavior. The reason for this, they say, is that inhaling certain scents alters brain waves and affects the pleasure center of the brain.

One study in particular investigated how aromatherapy can change an individual's mood. In this study, which was conducted in 2002 at the University of Southampton School of Medicine in England, fifteen extremely nervous psychiatric patients inhaled lavender oil for two hours a day every other day for ten days. On these days, 60 percent of the patients were reported to be calmer and happier. On the alternate days, however, when the patients inhaled a mist of pure water, there was no change in their mood.

Many acne patients report that aromatherapy has a similar effect on their response to stress. A former acne patient explains: "Even now, I still get an occasional acne breakout. It seems to happen most when I'm under stress at work. One of the ways I handle stress is by filling my oil lamp with lemon balm, and lighting it up right beside my hot tub. The combination of the warm bubbling water and the scented oil drains away my worries. No worries means no frown lines, and no pimples."[40]

Risks and Side Effects of Alternative Treatments

Although many people are turning to alternative treatments hoping to find safer forms of treatment, alternative treatments can also pose health risks. Vitamin B_5, for example, is known to cause iron deficiencies in some people. This can lead to serious health problems such as anemia. Other side effects of the vitamin include fatigue, weakness, dizziness, and dry skin that easily wounds.

Other problems occur due to lack of regulation of alternative products. Herbal products, in particular, can cause serious problems. Herbs can be as powerful as prescription drugs. But, unlike in prescription drugs, the level of active ingredients in herbal products and the dosage is not monitored by government agencies. Often, herbal products themselves, as well as the recommended dosages, are too strong for patients. But many people are unaware of this. They assume that because herbs are natural and have been used for thousands of years, these products are safe. However, high doses of certain herbs can cause nausea, stroke, heart problems, and hypersensitive skin. In addition, patients are just as likely to have an allergic reaction to herbs as to conventional medications. Moreover, scientists do not know what the long-term effect is of treatment with these products. This is a special problem when it comes to treatment with phytoestrogen. As yet, scientists do not know whether long-term phytoestrogen treatment, like conventional hormonal therapy, is linked to cancer and heart disease.

In addition, due to the lack of regulation, herbal products may contain herbs, chemicals, and drugs that are not listed on the label. For example, a 1999 random sampling in London, England, of eleven different herbal creams used to treat acne found that eight of the eleven products tested contained dexamethasone, a powerful steroid drug that was not listed on the labels. A 2003 article in *SKINmed*, a journal for dermatologists, explains:

> Guidelines concerning correct identification of the herb, the labeling of active ingredients, and establishment of purity are nonexistent. Lack of quality control too often leads to misidentification and contamination with toxic ingredients including pesticides, chemicals, heavy metals, and hidden drugs with their resultant ill effects. . . . From the reports of adverse reactions, it is becoming obvious that a history of traditional use is not a guarantee of safety.[41]

Yet these problems have not stopped millions of people with acne from turning to alternative treatments. "There are problems with every treatment," an acne patient explains. "Personally, I feel like natural treatments are gentler. Even if I'm wrong, when prescription products make your acne worse, and you can't look in the mirror without wanting to cry, you're willing to take a chance and try something different."[42]

Chapter 4

Living with Acne

PEOPLE WITH ACNE face a number of challenges that affect their daily lives. Acne care involves taking careful steps to improve, rather than worsen, acne symptoms as well as avoiding activities that can harm the skin. At the same time, people with acne must deal with emotional issues that acne can cause. Meeting these challenges helps people with acne lead happy lives.

Practicing Good Health Habits

One important thing people with acne must do in order to reduce their acne symptoms and lead happier lives is to practice good health habits. Although this is an important step for everyone to take, it is especially important for people with acne. For people with acne, practicing good health habits can keep bacteria from spreading, increase circulation and oxygen to the skin, help balance hormone levels, and reduce inflammation and infection.

Keeping the Skin Clean

Perhaps the most important good health habit that people with acne can practice is keeping their skin clean. Having clean skin keeps bacteria from spreading, reduces excess oil, and helps the skin shed dead cells. For acne patients this involves maintaining a delicate balance between cleansing the skin without irritating acne lesions, drying the skin, or spreading bacteria. This is accomplished through a carefully prescribed regimen that begins with gently washing the face no more than two to three times a day.

Although many people think that frequently scrubbing acne-infected areas stops acne outbreaks, this is not true. In fact, washing too often or using ordinary soaps can make the skin dry and sore, which worsens acne symptoms. Instead, acne patients use

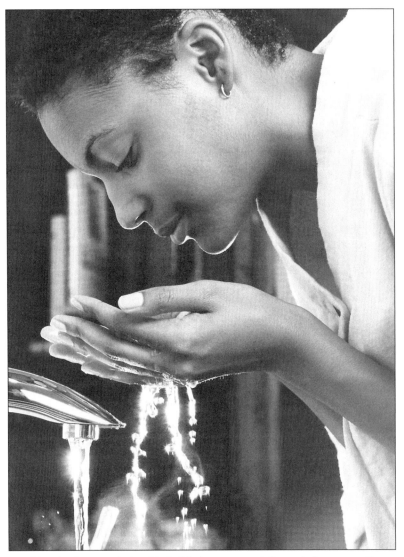

Washing the face regularly with facial cleansers specially made for acne sufferers can help improve a person's complexion.

mild facial cleansers, which are specially formulated not to irritate the skin. Ordinary soaps, on the other hand, contain harsh ingredients that can irritate inflamed acne lesions and dry out the skin. If the skin becomes too dry, the sebum glands overcompensate by producing even more oil, which exacerbates acne outbreaks.

Not only do acne patients use gentle soaps, they also use disposable washing pads or their fingers rather than a washcloth or loofah to cleanse acne-prone areas. The reason for this is that when a washcloth or loofah is used more than one time, it can trap and spread bacteria. In addition, washcloths and loofahs made from scratchy fabrics can irritate acne lesions and worsen inflammation. For the same reasons, acne patients use a fresh, clean, soft towel to gently pat, rather than rub, their skin dry once they are finished cleansing. Then, once acne patients have cleaned and dried their face, they can apply topical treatment. An acne patient recalls:

> When I first started breaking out, I scrubbed my face all the time with the same washcloth that hung in my bathroom for weeks, and the same soap that I scrubbed my hands with after I worked on my truck. Then I rubbed my face dry with the same towel I used on my hands. The only thing all that cleaning did was turn my blackheads into pusy red zits. Once the dermatologist straightened me out, I stopped using all that stuff, and my skin started to improve right away. [43]

Showers and Shampoo

People with acne must maintain the same delicate balance when they shower and shampoo their hair as they do in cleansing their faces. As with facial cleansers, acne patients use a specially formulated, gentle body cleanser when they shower, such as Dove or Oil of Olay body wash. This helps protect sensitive acne-prone areas of the body like the chest, back, and shoulders from being irritated.

Moreover, since many people with acne have oily hair, in order to keep oil from the hair from being transferred onto the forehead, neck, and back, where it can clog the pores and worsen acne outbreaks, people with acne must shampoo their hair every day. In addition, they must take special care to rinse their hair thoroughly. Otherwise, residue from shampoos or conditioners can clog the pores on a person's back and forehead. A young woman with acne explains how she solves this problem: "I have figured out how to keep my back and chest clear of zits: when you're in the shower, wash these areas with a gentle soap after you have rinsed the conditioner out of your hair. I know this can be a problem especially for girls with long hair; the conditioner goes down your back and leaves this nice zit-causing film that water doesn't wash off."[44]

Drinking Plenty of Water

In addition to using water to keep their skin clean, people with acne are advised to drink at least half their body weight in ounces of water each day. This means a one-hundred-pound individual should drink fifty ounces, or about seven glasses, of water a day.

Water carries waste material out of the body. This includes harmful chemicals, fats, and excess hormones. Without adequate water, the kidneys cannot produce enough urine to flush out wastes. Therefore, impurities that cannot be eliminated through urination are eliminated through the skin. This can cause toxins to build up in the pores, worsening acne outbreaks. In addition, without adequate water the liver, whose job it is to clear excess hormones out of the body, cannot function properly. As a result, excess hormones remain inside the body, where they stimulate the production of sebum and worsen acne. According to author and skin care expert Jennifer Thoden:

> Water . . . is quite possibly the single most important contributor to healing and preventing acne flare-ups. . . . If not enough water is consumed, toxins can build up causing breakouts. Water flushes these toxins out. . . . By drinking at least 8 glasses of water a day, you are flushing out the toxins that would normally escape through the pores of your skin . . . thus preventing acne breakouts.[45]

Getting Adequate Sleep

Another good health habit that is especially important for people with acne is getting adequate sleep. Sleep strengthens the body by allowing the body to rest, which in turn strengthens the immune system's ability to fight off acne-causing bacteria. It also helps regulate hormone production. A 1999 study at the University of Chicago Medical Center showed that cortisol production increases

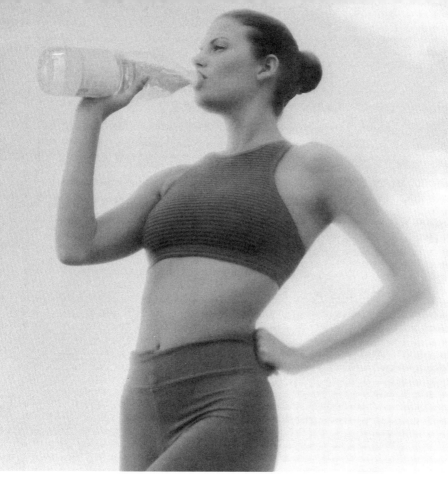

Drinking at least half of one's body weight in ounces of water each day prevents toxins and impurities from building up in the skin.

when people do not get adequate sleep. Since excess cortisol leads to increased sebum production, getting plenty of sleep keeps cortisol levels low and thus helps control acne.

In addition, a 2003 study conducted by the Endocrine Society in Chevy Chase, Maryland, found that a loss of just two hours of sleep per week increases the body's production of inflammation-causing chemicals by 60 percent. The result is a worsening of inflammatory acne. A former acne patient describes how lack of sleep affected his skin: "When I pulled an all-nighter my face erupted like a volcano; and not with little blackheads either, but with big red welts. As a teenager with acne I needed to get at least eight hours of sleep a night."[46]

While getting adequate sleep is important, acne outbreaks can be exacerbated if the bedding on which acne patients sleep is not changed often. When people sleep, oil, bacteria, and dead skin cells rub off their skin and accumulate on their bedding. The bedding absorbs these items, which then find their way back onto the skin, clogging the pores and causing new acne outbreaks. Therefore, it is important that people with acne change their sheets and pillowcases often. An acne patients explains: "I have found that changing my bedding, especially my pillowcase, every few days has helped my skin stay clear."[47]

Exercise

Exercise is another good health habit that helps improve acne symptoms. Besides being good for a person's overall health, exercise causes the body to release endorphins, natural chemicals

Regular exercise releases endorphins into the body that help relieve stress and stress-induced acne.

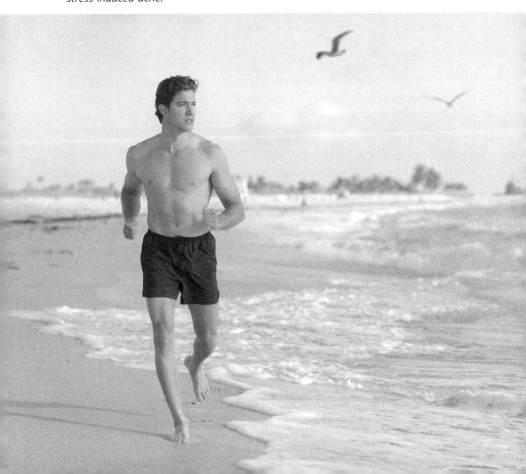

that give exercisers a feeling of well-being. This reduces stress and stress-induced acne outbreaks. For these reasons, it is important that people with acne get plenty of exercise.

As beneficial as exercise is, people with acne must take special care after they exercise to remove excess perspiration from their skin in order to prevent acne outbreaks. The reason for this is that perspiration can trap bacteria on the skin. If it is not washed off, the bacteria will eventually get trapped in hair follicles and aggravate acne symptoms. Tight-fitting athletic clothing can trap perspiration and rub and chafe the skin, which irritates and inflames acne lesions. Such garments as sweatbands, bicycle shorts, chin guards, and shoulder pads, to name a few, can exacerbate acne symptoms. Therefore, people with acne must take special care when they wear these types of garments and shower immediately after exercising to remove perspiration from their bodies.

Eating a Healthy Diet

Another good health habit that many people with acne practice is eating a healthy diet. Good nutrition helps the body to work properly. This is important in maintaining healthy skin. Eating a balanced diet high in vitamins, minerals, and fiber helps support the immune system and the body's ability to fight infection, including the bacteria that causes acne. Fiber found in fruits, vegetables, and cereal, in particular, helps the digestive system effectively eliminate waste. This keeps the body from eliminating waste through the skin, which can clog hair follicles.

Although specific foods have not been proven to cause acne, many scientists believe that certain foods may worsen acne symptoms. For instance, eating a diet high in linoleic acid, a fatty acid found in many fast foods and processed foods such as potato chips and donuts, may trigger the production of chemicals in the body that worsen inflammation. For this reason, people with acne are urged to limit their consumption of foods high in linoleic acid.

In addition, scientists have also linked foods high in iodine with increased acne outbreaks. For reasons that are yet unknown, the body cannot use excess iodine for energy. Nor can iodine be broken down effectively by the liver. Instead, it is excreted through the pores, where it can block hair follicles and cause irritation, inflammation, and worsening of acne symptoms.

Foods high in iodine include iodized salt, shellfish, and milk. In fact, a liter of milk contains anywhere from 450 to 1,000 micrograms of iodine, which gets into the milk through milking equipment and medication given to cows. According to Dr. James Fulton, the head of the Acne Research Institute in Newport Beach, California, "In some who are acne-prone, I'd say 1,000 micrograms or 1 milligram of iodine a day could be a problem."[48] Therefore, in order to reduce acne outbreaks, many people with acne avoid foods rich in iodine.

Avoiding Activities That Worsen Acne

Even when acne patients carefully practice good health habits, certain activities can worsen acne symptoms and should therefore be avoided. One such activity is squeezing acne lesions. Because acne lesions are filled with oil or pus, many acne patients think that they can reduce the size of a lesion and clear their skin by squeezing the oil and pus out of the lesion. However, this is not the case.

When acne lesions are squeezed, some oil and pus can be squeezed out. But at the same time, squeezing an acne lesion puts pressure on both the surface of the skin and the underlying layers. This pressure forces oil and bacteria deeper into the skin, leading to the formation of painful cysts. Moreover, squeezing the skin causes the skin to swell. Swelling puts pressure on the upper part of the hair follicles, which leads to the follicle becoming inflamed and the formation of new acne lesions.

Worse still, squeezing acne lesions damages skin tissue, and in the case of cysts, causes them to break and bleed. The result is a scar that forms where the skin tissue was damaged or the cyst was broken. Los Angeles skin care expert Arcona Devan warns her clients: "Don't pick at your skin. It's one of the worst things you can do. Squeezing blemishes injures your skin and can create scars."[49]

Keeping the Hands off the Face

Even when individuals with acne refrain from squeezing acne lesions, unless they are careful to keep their hands off their faces,

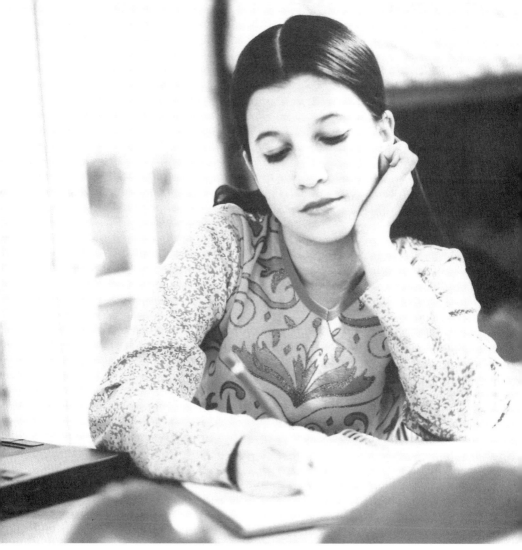

Acne sufferers who touch their faces with their hands can exacerbate their acne because even clean hands transmit bacteria.

acne symptoms can worsen. Unwashed hands hold bacteria that can easily spread from the hands to the face. Even clean hands can spread bacteria when they touch bacteria-infected acne lesions. The bacteria is transferred onto the hands and then onto the face or body. Because many people habitually rest their chins on their hands, people with acne must make a conscious effort to avoid doing this. A young man explains: "When the dermatologist told me to keep my hands off my face, I had to work at it. I was surprised how often I touched my face. It's not something you think about until the doctor tells you to. It's not easy to stop either. But I don't want new zits all over my face, so I really watch myself."[50]

Avoiding Oil-Based Cosmetics

Just as touching the face can worsen acne symptoms, so can using makeup that contains oil. Lanolin, petroleum jelly, and other oils in oil-based makeup can clog the pores, causing acne outbreaks. Even lipsticks with moisturizers and hair products such as gel and mousse can clog the pores along the lip line and forehead, respectively. Since many people with acne use cosmetics to conceal acne lesions, the oil in these products can be a problem. Therefore, in an effort to hide acne blemishes without worsening their acne, many acne patients use specially labeled, water-based, noncomedogenic makeup. Unlike oil-based makeup, such makeup does not clog the pores. And, in order to keep from spreading oil and bacteria, acne patients should wash their makeup brushes and sponges often.

Unfortunately, even noncomedogenic products sometimes contain a small amount of oil that makes the product easier to apply. This can aggravate acne outbreaks in some patients. In order to test how much oil is in a product, many acne patients place a dab of makeup on a piece of white paper and wait to see if an oil ring forms. The larger the oil ring, the more oil in the product. Many acne patients report being surprised by the size of the oil ring that many popular cosmetics form. But by doing the test, acne patients learn which products they should avoid.

When patients switch from oil-based cosmetics to water-based products, they are usually quite happy with the results. They report water-based cosmetics work well at concealing their complexion flaws and cause fewer acne outbreaks. Beauty and skin care expert Bobbi Brown agrees. "Don't even think of wearing anything except an oil-free [makeup] formula,"[51] she advises her clients with acne.

Taking Special Care When Shaving

Shaving can also worsen acne. Razors can cut acne lesions, causing pustules and cysts to rupture. If the cutting edge of the razor is not clean, it can spread bacteria and oil. If it is not sharp, it can irritate the skin and cause a razor burn, which makes the skin appear redder than usual.

In particular, shaving with a dry razor causes problems. Washing the face before shaving softens the skin and beard. Conversely, when the face is dry, the shaver's skin and beard are tough. Therefore, the shaver must apply more pressure to the razor in order to remove facial hair. This irritates the skin and leads to razor burn.

Dull or dry razors can cut acne lesions and spread bacteria. Men with acne should use sharp, wet razors when shaving.

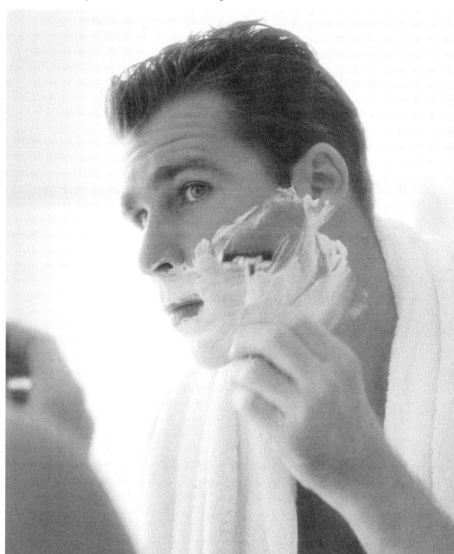

Consequently, most men with acne use a wet razor or an electric razor, which requires even less pressure than a wet razor and is thus gentler on the skin.

Shaving lotions can also cause problems. Lotions that are not noncomedogenic can clog pores just as cosmetics can, and after-shave lotions that contain alcohol can dry out the skin and cause an increase in sebum production. In fact, because shaving and shaving products present so many problems for men with acne, many male acne patients try to avoid shaving whenever they can. A former acne patient explains: "I've had some bad experiences shaving, like burning my face and turning it bright red, and slicing open my pimples. Some of the scars I have are from pimples I destroyed shaving. Even now, I try not to shave every day. I still get little pimples, and shaving is hard on my skin. When I do shave, I use an electric razor, and I don't press hard."[52]

Avoiding Unhealthy Environments

Just as people with acne avoid shaving with a dry razor, they also often avoid certain environments that can worsen acne symptoms. Oil in the air in the kitchen of a fast-food restaurant or in a gas station, for example, can settle on the skin of acne patients and clog hair follicles, causing acne outbreaks. For this reason, many people with acne avoid working where they come in contact with oil in the air.

Hot, humid environments, which cause people to perspire excessively, also exacerbate acne symptoms by causing perspiration that traps bacteria on the skin. Indeed, many acne patients report increased acne outbreaks when they travel to hot, humid places on vacation. Consequently, they often choose to vacation in cooler, drier environments. Many people with acne who live in hot, humid environments try to stay indoors in an air-conditioned environment as much as possible. When they do go outdoors, they take special care to remove excess perspiration from their skin as quickly as possible.

Sunlight can also cause problems for people with acne. Although sunlight helps dry out oily skin, for patients who are using Accutane, antibiotics, or retinoids, exposure to sunlight can be dangerous. Many acne medicines cause photosensitivity, which makes the skin burn easily when it is exposed to sunlight. Therefore, many people with acne avoid exposure to sunlight.

Coping with Emotional Issues

While people with acne should avoid certain activities and environments and practice good health habits to improve the physical symptoms of acne, they also must deal with the emotional issues caused by acne in order to lead happier lives. One such issue is low self-esteem. Talking with a counselor or a psychologist helps acne patients recognize why they suffer from low self-esteem and investigate ways to change or avoid these feelings. An acne patient describes how talking to a counselor helped her. "Before I started seeing him [the counselor], I hated the person I saw in the mirror. He helped me realize that there is more to me than my appearance. I'm smart and funny. I realize the person in the mirror isn't all I am. Because of what I learned in counseling, I'm a happier person, and I feel better about myself."[53]

Staying Active

Another way acne patients deal with emotional issues is by staying active. Getting involved in activities that are fun and that focus on others helps people with acne to forget about their appearance while raising their self-esteem. Supporting a cause, joining a club or church group, or doing volunteer work are a few of the ways people with acne stay active and raise their self-esteem in the process. A former acne patient explains:

> Being a teenager with pimples, that was bad. I knew I wasn't popular. I knew I wasn't attractive to girls. There was a lot of anger and humiliation. I wanted to avoid social activities and stay home and hide. But I went out anyway. I had to get over myself. I had to put myself out there, pimples and all. One of the things I did was volunteer at the animal shelter. The animals didn't care how I looked. They licked my face, welts and

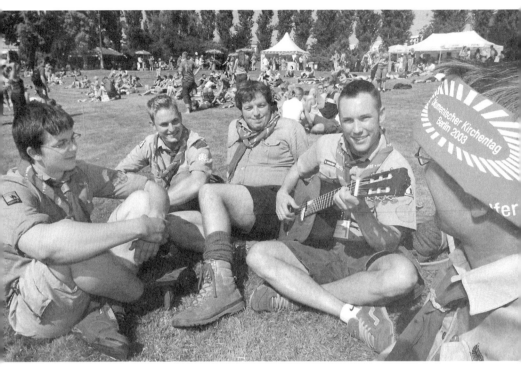

Participating in activities like this church group picnic can raise the self-esteem of acne sufferers and help them deal with emotional issues.

all. After a while I didn't care either. I was doing something that made me feel good inside. That made me look better outside.[54]

It is clear that people with acne face many challenges. But by dealing with emotional issues and carefully protecting and caring for their skin, they can meet these challenges and live happy, productive lives.

Chapter 5

What the Future Holds

S INCE ACNE TREATMENTS are not always effective and can cause serious side effects, scientists are focusing their research on developing safer and more effective acne treatments. In an effort to do this, they are concentrating on learning more about hormonal changes and the bacteria that are linked to acne. At the same time, scientists are developing less invasive treatments to minimize acne scars.

Studying Hormonal Changes

Because hormonal changes are closely linked to sebum production, scientists are trying to determine whether acne flare-ups are linked to a specific time in a woman's menstrual cycle. Although doctors and patients have frequently reported the occurrence of acne flare-ups in the week before a patient's menstrual period, this link has never been formally studied. In an effort to investigate this link, in 2001 scientists in Downstate Medical Center in Brooklyn, New York, conducted a study of four hundred female acne patients aged twelve to fifty-two. The women were asked whether their acne appeared to be related to their menstrual period, and if so, whether it worsened before, during, or after their menstrual period. Forty-four percent of the women reported an increase in acne flare-ups in the week before their menstrual period. According to the survey's director, Dr. Alan R. Shalita: "Acne has often been associated with hormones and a woman's monthly cycle. This study confirms that many women do, indeed, have a premenstrual flare of their acne."[55]

In fact, similar results were found in a 1973 British study that examined the relationship between sebum duct openings and a woman's menstrual cycle. The openings, the study showed, were enlarged and produced the most oil between the twenty-first and twenty-sixth day of a twenty-eight-day menstrual cycle. On an average, the study found that the greatest amount of oil production and accompanying acne outbreaks were most likely to occur on the twenty-second day of the cycle.

Although the results of the 2001 study appear to verify the 1973 study, scientists are continuing their research in this area because the 1973 study was a small, isolated study that was not followed up by similar studies. However, based on the results of the 1973 and 2001 studies, many patients are tracking their menstrual cycles, and their doctors are strengthening their acne treatments during the time of the month when flare-ups are most likely to occur. The results have been heartening. Shalita explains: "Acne that worsens during a woman's monthly cycle isn't something that women will grow out of as they get older. Seeing your dermatologist to determine the best treatment plan for acne flare-ups is recommended for successful results."[56]

Learning About the Bacteria That Cause Acne

While some scientists are investigating the link between hormonal changes and acne, others are studying the bacteria that cause infected acne lesions. Through laboratory studies, scientists have identified a bacterium known as Propionibacterium acnes as the primary cause of infected acne lesions. By learning more about this bacterium, scientists hope to develop new ways to combat it.

Using the Bacterium's Genome to Develop a Vaccine

One way scientists hope to learn more about Propionibacterium acnes is by studying its genome, or genetic structure. In 2001 scientists in Seattle successfully decoded the genome of Propionibacterium acnes. Through laboratory studies, scientists have determined that Propionibacterium acnes is composed of 2.8 million DNA pairs, and they have determined the exact order of the pairs. Using this infor-

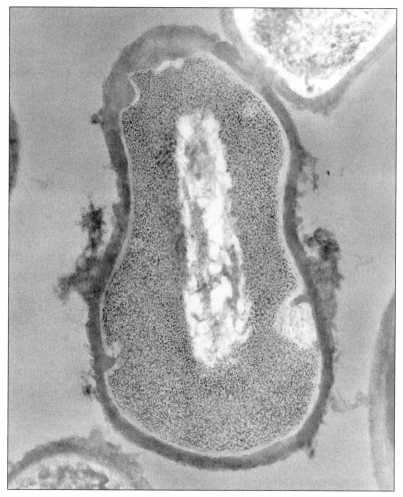

As scientists study the bacterium responsible for acne, Propionibacterium acnes (pictured), they search for innovative ways to combat the disease.

mation, scientists hope to develop a vaccine made of microorganisms known as antigens that would attack the DNA pairs that form Propionibacterium acnes. This attack, scientists theorize, would so weaken the DNA pairs that they would separate. This would upset the order of the DNA chain that forms Propionibacterium acnes, killing or at least weakening the bacterium.

Although this vaccine would not stop a person's hair follicles from becoming clogged, thus preventing comedones from developing, it would reduce infection in pustules and cysts and prevent papules from becoming infected. Such a vaccine, scientists think, would be a more effective way to treat acne with less serious side effects than many existing treatments. Unfortunately, scientists have not yet identified a group of antigens capable of separating the DNA pairs that form Propionibacterium acnes. According to Steven Gillis, chairman of the study: "This is not something that we're going to file for registration on [get permission from the FDA to place on the market] tomorrow. But it's a very novel approach to a major medical problem. . . . Our goal is now to identify the antigens that might be combined to be part of a vaccine. . . . It certainly holds some promise for the future."[57]

A Vaccine to Counter Heat-Shock Proteins

Other scientists at the University of Leeds in England are taking a different approach. They are investigating how another group of proteins, called heat-shock proteins, worsen inflammation. Heat-shock proteins are found in all bacteria, including Propionibacterium acnes. Scientists theorize that heat produced by these proteins stresses and overstimulates the immune system. This, according to the theory, incites the immune system to flood the area around Propionibacterium acnes with infection-fighting chemicals. As a result, excess chemicals spill over and attack surrounding healthy skin cells, which increases the inflammation of acne lesions and spreads inflammation to surrounding skin. Making matters worse, scientists say, once an attack is mounted, the stress of the attack causes Propionibacterium acnes to produce even more heat-shock protein. This causes the cycle to repeat and acne lesions to become even more inflamed. According to researcher Dr. Mark Farrar: "Under stress, the bacteria may produce more heat-shock protein, and these can induce strong immune responses. If the immune system does not distinguish between the human and bacterial proteins, it may attack healthy cells and so contribute to inflammation."[58]

In an effort to counter the effect of heat-shock protein on acne lesions, scientists are trying to develop a vaccine that would minimize the effect the protein has on the immune system. Such a vaccine could prevent or even cure inflamed and cystic acne. However, since scientists do not as yet know what type of substance inhibits the heat-shock protein, it may be years before such a vaccine is developed. Leeds University professor Eileen Ingham explains: "If the heat shock proteins are shown to be the major cause of inflammation, children could be vaccinated before they reach puberty, to help them develop a regulated response to the proteins and to reduce the chances of the condition [acne] occurring."[59]

Because heat-shock proteins like this exacerbate acne inflammation, scientists are developing a vaccine that will inhibit such proteins and prevent or cure cystic acne.

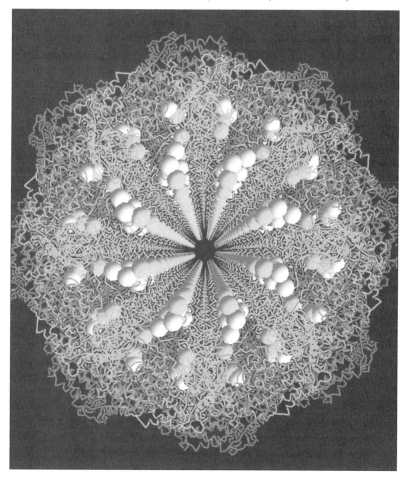

Using a Virus to Fight the Bacterium

Since the development of a vaccine for acne is still far in the future, some scientists are taking a different approach. They are combining what they know about Propionibacterium acnes with the study of bacteriophages, viruses that are deadly to bacteria but harmless to humans. When a bacterium is exposed to a deadly bacteriophage, the bacteriophage attaches itself to the cell wall surrounding the bacterium. Since the sole goal of any virus is to reproduce, once the bacteriophage attaches itself to the cell wall, it injects its own DNA into the bacterium and begins replicating itself. This causes millions of viruses to be produced inside the bacterium. The viruses continuously reproduce until they cause the bacterium to burst and be destroyed. From here, the viruses enter the bloodstream, where they themselves are destroyed by the immune system. Since specific bacteriophages attack specific bacteria, scientists hope to identify and isolate a bacteriophage that targets Propi-

A technician takes inventory of crates of zinc at a factory. Zinc contains antibacterial properties that could help in fighting acne bacteria.

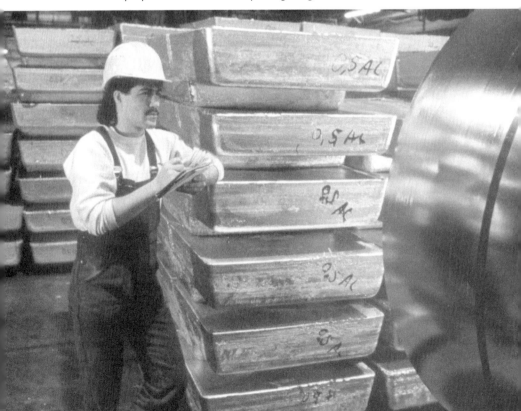

onibacterium acnes. Once such a bacteriophage is identified, scientists hope to use it in a topical treatment that could be rubbed directly on infected acne lesions, killing the underlying bacteria on contact. Although scientists have discovered a bacteriophage that attacks the streptococcus bacterium that causes strep throat and the flesh-eating disease, they have not yet discovered one that targets Propionibacterium acnes. Therefore, research is ongoing.

Combining Zinc and Antibiotics

While some scientists are working on developing a topical treatment made from a bacteriophage, other scientists are trying to pinpoint whether there may be certain vitamins or minerals that, when combined with antibiotics, would effectively combat Propionibacterium acnes. This has led scientists at Leeds University, England, to develop a new gel that combines the mineral zinc with the antibiotic drug clindamycin.

Scientists theorize that zinc, which is found in foods such as beans and artichokes, stimulates the immune system to produce bacteria-fighting white blood cells and, when it is applied to an infected area, has antibacterial properties that destroy bacteria. Therefore, combining zinc in a topical gel with a traditional antibiotic used to treat acne, such as clindamycin, helps to increase the treatment's potency. The increased strength of the treatment allows acne patients to apply the combination gel only once a day, instead of at least twice a day as with other topical treatments. Since it is applied less frequently, this treatment causes less redness and irritation than more frequent applications of topical treatments.

To discover whether the gel, known as Zindacellin, is more potent than simple antibiotic gels, a clinical trial was held in 2002 in Leeds in which 240 people with mild to moderate acne applied the combination gel once a day for eight weeks. At the same time another group applied a topical clindamycin gel twice a day. The results showed that a once-daily application of Zindacellin was at least, if not more, effective than twice daily applications of clindamycin. According to dermatology professor William Cunliffe, who conducted the trials: "This is a new preparation aimed at concentrating the drug in the skin so it will then last for twenty-four hours. . . . The zinc is there to maintain the concentration of the drug. It also works as an anti-microbial, reducing the bugs [bacteria] in acne. . . . If you use it just once a day, you are going to have less irritation in the long term."[60]

Other trials are being conducted throughout England. So far, patients and scientists are hopeful. A young woman who is participating in one trial explains: "I didn't notice the improvement at the beginning, but I have in the past three or four weeks. The last time I saw my doctor, he said there had been a big improvement, and I'm hoping if I keep it up it'll completely clear my skin."[61]

Using Heat to Destroy the Bacteria

Scientists in New York are exploring another angle. They are using heat in the form of high-intensity light to combat Propionibacterium acnes. One new treatment that was approved by the FDA in the fall of 2002 uses a high-intensity blue light known as Clearlight. During treatment with Clearlight, patients lie on a machine similar to a tanning bed from which a harmless, blue light pulsates. The light stimulates Propionibacterium acnes to produce a chemical called porphyrin, which attacks the bacterium and causes it to self-destruct. Scientists are unsure why this occurs. However, the results have been excellent. For example, in a 2002 study at Downstate Medical Center in Brooklyn, New York, acne patients who were treated with Clearlight twice a week for four weeks showed a 60 percent decrease in visible acne lesions with no side effects. Consequently, Clearlight is believed to be as effective, and gentler, on the body than antibiotics and other oral acne medicine. A patient who was treated with Clearlight talks about the results: "They're really good. I haven't broken out since I've taken the treatment. I'm not as self-conscious as I was before. My face is basically clear."[62]

In a similar manner, scientists are using heat in radio waves to destroy Propionibacterium acnes. In this procedure, doctors run a hand-held treatment probe over the patient's skin. The probe releases a cool spray of ice and chemicals that numb and protect the skin. At the same time, the probe releases radio waves that generate heat and penetrate deep below the surface of the skin. The heat shrinks the skin and the oil glands. This makes wrinkles and acne scars appear smaller and decreases the flow of oil and the development of acne lesions. A number of studies have reported treatment with radio waves to be effective in eliminating acne lesions and making acne scars less visible. Therefore, the FDA approved the use of ThermaCool TC, one type of radio wave acne treatment, in 2003.

Using Lasers to Minimize Pitted Acne Scars

Because heat in blue light and radio waves has proven so effective in treating acne, scientists are investigating using heat in the form of lasers to develop less invasive ways to minimize pitted acne scars. In fact, one treatment known as CO_2 laser resurfacing has been in use since the late 1990s. In addition, a newer, more effective process called super-pulsed CO_2 laser resurfacing has recently been developed. Both processes use an instrument that looks like a crane arm with a laser pointer attached to the end. The pointer emits an invisible carbon dioxide–based laser beam that vaporizes the outer layer of a person's skin. Since the skin rejuvenates, damaging the top layer of a person's skin causes healthier skin cells under the skin's surface to grow and gradually replace the damaged skin. The new skin fills in the depressions that form pitted scars, making them appear less obvious.

Unfortunately, most acne scars affect more than one layer of skin, and the CO_2 laser, which emits only one laser beam, can reach only one layer. This is why the super-pulsed laser was developed. It emits a number of laser beams of differing wavelengths that can reach any number of skin layers. This allows the doctor to selectively target the depth of the skin area to vaporize and to remove more skin when needed with increased accuracy and control.

Although less invasive than traditional skin dermabrasion surgery, both super-pulsed and CO_2 laser resurfacing take from one to three hours to administer and require that the patient be sedated. And, because the skin is burned, it often oozes, peels, and appears red for several weeks after the procedure. In addition, since super-pulsed CO_2 laser resurfacing frequently targets underlying layers of skin, it can vaporize irreplaceable skin cells

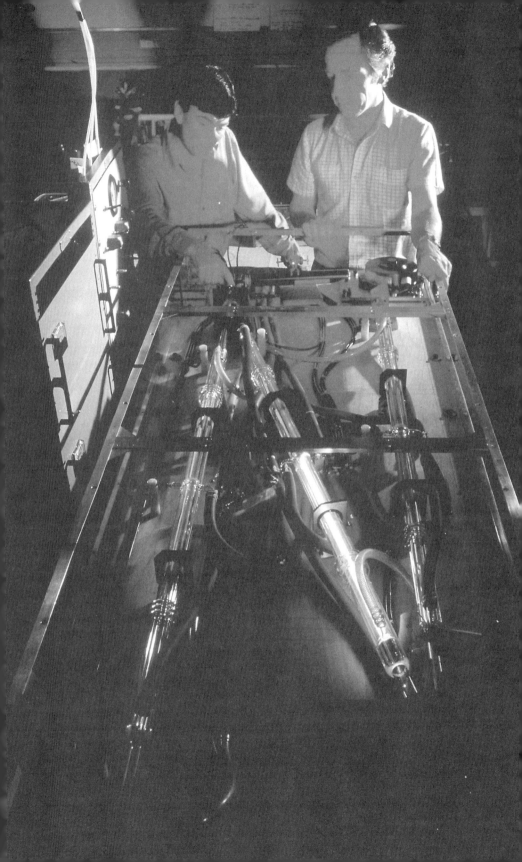

that produce pigment. Without adequate pigment, the skin loses its color. This can be a problem for dark-skinned people whose skin may be left with permanent white blotches. Moreover, this type of treatment does not work for keloid scars. Scientists say that people whose skin develops keloid scars from acne damage tend to form keloid scars for other types of skin damage as well. Since super-pulsed and CO_2 laser resurfacing damages the skin, these people are likely to form keloid scars as a response to the treatment. Therefore, super-pulsed and CO_2 laser resurfacing is not for everyone. Despite the disadvantages, according to experts at the Loftus Plastic Surgery Center in Cincinnati, Ohio, people who undergo either procedure are generally happy with the results. Most report a 30 percent improvement in the appearance of their acne scars.

Because of the problems associated with super-pulsed and CO_2 laser resurfacing, scientists are developing a newer laser treatment known as YAG. YAG promises to be less invasive and require less recovery time than either type of CO_2 laser treatment. YAG uses an instrument similar to that used to administer super-pulsed CO_2 laser resurfacing. But with YAG, the instrument delivers a cool, numbing spray to the surface of the skin in combination with an infrared laser beam that the doctor aims directly at the patient's acne scars. The infrared beam does not affect the surface of the skin. Instead, it penetrates deep beneath the skin, where it shrinks skin cells. This causes the body to produce increased amounts of collagen to rebuild the shrunken skin cells. Abundant collagen not only rebuilds the skin cells, but also cushions and plumps up the surface layer of skin, giving it a smoother appearance and raising and filling in pitted acne scars.

Scientists report good results in studies in which YAG laser treatment has been used. In a 2001 study conducted at the University of California in San Diego, fourteen subjects with pitted acne scars were treated with YAG laser for twelve weeks. By the

Scientists test a CO_2 laser. CO_2 laser resurfacing uses a carbon dioxide–based laser beam to burn away skin with acne and minimize pitted scars.

end of the last treatment all the subjects showed a 40 percent improvement in the appearance of their acne scars. Improvement was measured by how much each pitted acne scar was raised after treatment.

YAG treatment is reported to be relatively painless. Patients say it feels like a rubber band being snapped across their skin. More importantly, results from YAG treatment are reported to last for years, and the treatment does not create any visible wounds or redness of the skin. In addition, because it does not vaporize underlying skin cells, it does not lighten the skin. Dr. Mitchel Goldman, who conducted the 2001 San Diego study, explains:

> YAG laser is an excellent method for treating acne scars because it works for all skin types—from very dark to very light—and with no down time. Until now, many of the other acne scar treatments produced a wound that may have required weeks to heal. Since this new laser therapy is non-invasive, the patient does not require anesthesia and the procedure is not a painful one.[63]

Filling in Acne Scars with Fat

Although super-pulsed CO_2 laser resurfacing and YAG penetrate deep below the surface of the skin, neither of these treatments can penetrate deep enough or produce enough collagen or new skin cells to correct the deepest, most severe type of acne scars. Consequently, scientists have developed a way to minimize these scars by using a patient's own body fat to fill in the scars in a process called autologous fat transfer. Autologous fat transfer involves transferring a patient's own body fat from one area of his or her body to another. The fat is generally extracted from the hips, buttocks, or abdomen after the area is numbed and a small incision is made. Then, a syringe with a long, thin tube attached is inserted into the area. Fat is suctioned through the tube and transferred to a sterile flask, where it is washed free of oil, anesthetic, and blood. Then the fat is injected in small quantities below the surface of the skin of pitted acne scars. The fat fills in the depressed

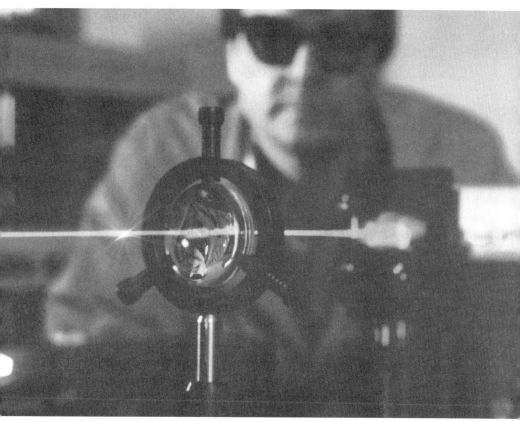

A technician monitors a YAG laser. Treatment with YAG lasers is less invasive and requires less recovery time than CO_2 laser treatment.

part of the scar, minimizing its appearance. In order to fill in multiple or deeply pitted acne scars, multiple syringes are usually used. However, over time fat starts to break down and some of the transplanted fat eventually is reabsorbed into the skin. This means that in about six to eighteen months, acne scars will once again reappear, and the procedure must be repeated.

Since repeated autologous fat transfers can be uncomfortable, scientists are experimenting with substances other than a patient's own body fat to use in this process. So far, they have developed a way to substitute bovine collagen, or collagen extracted from cows, for a patient's own fat. However, since the immune system identifies the bovine collagen as a foreign object, it usually is destroyed by the immune system in three to six months. Moreover, many patients have an allergic reaction to bovine collagen. Therefore, scientists are continuing to work on developing a long-lasting substance that will not cause any side effects. This includes experiments with the plastic Gore-Tex, which so far scientists have been unable to produce in injectable form.

Scientists have also been experimenting with skin tissue derived from human sources. Sheets of skin are donated to tissue banks in the same way as organs such as livers or hearts are donated. Then, the sheets of skin undergo a process in which they are turned into an injectable semiliquid or powdered form, which is administered in the same manner as autologous fat. Since skin naturally regenerates, the newly injected skin quickly repopulates the injected area, causing depressed acne scars to fill in.

This procedure has been available to patients since 2000. At first, scientists thought it would offer patients a permanent solution to minimizing acne scars. However, transferred skin tissue, like bovine collagen, is targeted by the immune system as a foreign object and is broken down by the immune system in three to six months. Therefore, scientists are still working on perfecting this procedure in order to make it longer lasting.

Although scientists have not yet discovered a way to permanently erase acne scars, there is optimism that such a discovery is on the horizon. There are many ongoing studies investigating hormonal changes and Propionibacterium acnes, and with the development of new, safer, more effective, and less invasive treatments, the future looks bright for people with acne. Indeed, a cure may be found in the future, but for now, new treatments give people with acne hope.

Notes

Introduction: A Disease That Is Often Ignored
1. Fred [pseud.], interview with the author, Dallas, Texas, May 15, 2003.
2. Quoted in Tamar Nordenberg, "Battling Blemishes and Beyond," Discovery Health Channel. www.health.discovery.com.
3. Fred, interview.
4. Quoted in Linda Papadopoulous and Carl Walker, *Understanding Skin Problems.* West Sussex, England: Wiley, 2003, p. 16.
5. Quoted in Anthony C. Chu and Anne Lovell, *The Good Skin Doctor.* London: HarperCollins, 1999, p. 129.
6. Fred, interview.

Chapter 1: What Is Acne?
7. Mike [pseud.], interview with the author, Dallas, Texas, May 16, 2003.
8. Fred, interview.
9. Fred, interview.
10. Fred, interview.
11. Fred, interview.
12. Chu and Lovell, *The Good Skin Doctor,* p. 15.
13. Quoted in Acne.org, "Success Stories." www.acne.org.
14. Chu and Lovell, *The Good Skin Doctor,* p. 81.
15. Quoted in American Academy of Dermatology, "The Social Impact of Acne." www.derm-infonet.com.
16. Quoted in Acne Support Group, "Top Ten Problems." www.stop spots.org.
17. Quoted in Acne.org, "Success Stories."
18. Fred, interview.

Chapter 2: Diagnosis and Treatment

19. Quoted in Julia Necheff, "Emotional Scars from Acne Linger," *Canadian Press,* September 2, 1999. www.slam.ca.
20. Richard [pseud.], interview with the author, Dallas, Texas, May 27, 2003.
21. Quoted in Acne.org, "Success Stories."
22. Quoted in Acne Net, "Acne Net Update." www.skincarephy sicians.com.
23. Fred, interview.
24. Rachel [pseud.], interview with the author, Las Cruces, New Mexico, June 14, 2003.
25. Chu and Lovell, *The Good Skin Doctor,* p. 62.
26. Quoted in Acne.org, "Accutane." www.acne.org.
27. Quoted in Acne.org, "Success Stories."
28. "Bleeding Misery of the Boy Cursed by a Common Cure," *Australian,* January 18, 2003. http://searchepnet.com.
29. Quoted in Acne.org, "Success Stories."
30. Quoted in Katherine Hobson, "Mind Versus Face," *U.S. News & World Report,* April 1, 2002, p. 61.
31. Quoted in Necheff, "Emotional Scars from Acne Linger."
32. Fred, interview.

Chapter 3: Alternative and Complementary Treatments

33. Brittney [pseud.], interview with the author, Las Cruces, New Mexico, June 18, 2003.
34. Quoted in Gale Maleskey, *Nature's Medicines.* Emmaus, PA: Rodale Press, 1999, p. 98.
35. Quoted in Chu and Lovell, *The Good Skin Doctor,* p. 72.
36. Quoted in Coenzyme-A Technologies Inc., "Testimonials for Clear Skin Image." www.coenzyme-a.com.
37. Quoted in Clare Le Dor.Com, "Clare Lé Dor Natural Acne Treatment System." www.clareledor.com.
38. Palle Rosted, "Treatment of Skin Diseases with Acupuncture—A Review," The Medical Acupuncture Web Page. http://users.med.auth.gr.
39. Brittney, interview.
40. Rachel, interview.
41. Joseph A. Witkowski and Lawrence Charles Parish, "Dermatologic Manifestations of Complementary Therapy," *SKINmed,* 2003, p. 175.

42. Brittney, interview.

Chapter 4: Living with Acne
43. Mike, interview.
44. Quoted in Chaos Kids, "Juicy Zits." http://chaoskids.com.
45. Jennifer Thoden, "How Eight Glasses of Water a Day Can Keep Acne Away," About Holistic Healing. www.healing.about.com.
46. Fred, interview.
47. Quoted in Exposed, "Tips." www.exposedskincare.com.
48. Quoted in Hungerstrike.com, "Got Zits?" www.hungerstrike.com.
49. Quoted in "Beauty Talk," *In Style*, July 2003, p. 146.
50. Mike, interview.
51. Bobby Brown and Sally Wadyka, *Beauty Evolution.* New York: HarperResource, 2002, p. 102.
52. Fred, interview.
53. Brittney, interview.
54. Fred, interview.

Chapter 5: What the Future Holds
55. Quoted in American Academy of Dermatology, "Study Confirms Monthly Hormonal Changes in Menstrual Cycle Affect Acne Flare-Ups." www.aad.org.
56. Quoted in American Academy of Dermatology, "Study Confirms Monthly Hormonal Changes in Menstrual Cycle Affect Acne Flare-Ups."
57. Quoted in Marni Leff, "Acne Vaccine May Be on the Horizon," *Seattle Post-Intelligencer,* April 6, 2001. http://seattlepi.nwsource.com.
58. Quoted in Anjana Ahuja, "Could a Jab Cure Teenage Spots?" *Times* (London), November 5, 2001, p. 17.
59. Quoted in Ahuja, "Could a Jab Cure Teenage Spots?"
60. Quoted in Rory Clements, "The Once a Day Gel That Can Beat Acne," *Daily Mail* (London), March 19, 2002. http://search.epnet.com.
61. Quoted in Clements, "The Once a Day Gel That Can Beat Acne."
62. Quoted in Curelight.com, "CureLight on NBC Health Watch (February 18, 2003)." www.curelight.com.
63. Quoted in American Academy of Dermatology, "Study Finds New Laser Treatment Helps Heal the Physical and Emotional Scars of Acne." www.aad.org.

Glossary

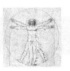

Accutane: A popular drug used to treat severe acne. It is also known as isotretinoin.

acne: A common skin disease.

androgen: A male sex hormone produced by both men and women.

bacteriophage: A virus that is deadly to bacteria but harmless to humans.

benzoyl peroxide: A topical treatment for acne.

collagen: A natural substance that helps the skin regenerate.

comedones: Acne lesions that appear in the form of whiteheads and blackheads.

cysts: Large, inflamed acne lesions occurring deep under the skin.

dermatologist: A doctor who specializes in diseases of the skin.

estrogen: A female sex hormone.

follicles: Tiny ducts in the skin where hair grows.

genome: All the genes in an organism.

heat-shock protein: Cellular protein that stimulates inflammation.

hormones: A variety of chemicals produced by the body to regulate different body functions.

ice-pick or pitted scars: Acne scars that are caused by tissue loss.

inflammation: Redness, swelling, and heat produced by the immune system to combat infection.

isotretinoin: A powerful drug derived from vitamin A that is used to treat severe acne.

keloid scars: Acne scars that form as a result of increased tissue formation.

noncomedogenic: Cosmetics that do not contain oil and will not clog pores.

papules: Red, mildly inflamed acne lesions.

phytoestrogen: A plant-based female hormone–like compound that increases the effect of the female sex hormone, estrogen.

pores: Tiny openings in the skin.

porphyrin: A chemical that attacks and kills acne-causing bacteria.

Propionibacterium acnes: The bacterium that causes infected acne lesions.

pustules: Large, pus-filled acne lesions.

salicylic acid: A topical treatment used to treat comedones.

sebaceous gland: The gland that produces sebum.

sebum: A natural oil the body produces to protect and moisten the skin.

skin dermabrasion: A surgical treatment used to reduce acne scars.

testosterone: A male sex hormone.

topical treatments: Medications that are applied directly onto the skin.

Organizations to Contact

American Academy of Dermatology
PO Box 4014
Schaumburg, IL 60168-4014
(888) 462-3376
fax: (847) 330-0050
www.aad.org
The American Academy of Dermatology publishes brochures and fact sheets on acne and offers referrals to dermatologists and information on every aspect of acne.

Association for Dermatologic Surgery
5550 Meadowbrook Dr., Suite 120
Rolling Meadows, IL 60008
(847) 956-0900
www.aboutskinsurgery.com
The Association for Dermatologic Surgery offers information on skin surgery, including surgery for acne scars, and news updates on the latest research developments in skin surgery.

National Center for Complementary and Alternative Medicine Clearinghouse
PO Box 8218
Silver Spring, MD 20907-8218
(888) 644-6226
http://altmed.od.nih.gov
This organization provides information and conducts research on the effectiveness of alternative treatments.

**National Institute of Arthritis and Musculoskeletal
and Skin Diseases**
1 AMS Circle
Bethesda, MD 20892-3675
(877) 226-4267
fax: (301) 718-6366
www.niams.nih.gov

This organization provides information about various diseases, including acne.

For Further Reading

Books

Jennifer Ceasar, *Everything You Need to Know About Acne: A Helping Book for Teens.* New York: Rosen Publishing, 2000. An easy-to-read book that exams the causes, treatments, and myths surrounding acne.

Terry J. Dubrow and Brenda D. Adderly, *The Acne Cure.* Emmaus, PA: Rodale Press, 2003. Maps out a nonprescription treatment plan for acne.

Erika Lutz, *The Complete Idiot's Guide to Looking Great for Teens.* Indianapolis: Alpha Books, 2001. Gives tips on looking good, including facts on acne and skin care.

Websites

Acne Net (www.skincarephysicians.com). An educational website maintained by the American Academy of Dermatology that provides information on every aspect of acne, including help in finding a dermatologist.

Acne.org (www.acne.org). Offers a wealth of information about acne as well as online support and chat groups.

Acne Support Group (www.stopspots.org). Based in England, this is the largest acne support group in the world. It provides information, relaxation tapes, and online support.

American Academy of Dermatology (www.aad.org). Provides a wealth of information about every aspect of acne, including news on the latest research.

Chaos Kids (http://chaoskids.com). A website that features humorous true stories and advice by acne sufferers about their skin problems.

Facefacts (www.facefacts.com). Provides information about Accutane, information on managing acne, acne myths and facts, and treatment success stories.

Works Consulted

Books

Bobbi Brown and Sally Wadyka, *Beauty Evolution.* New York: Harper-Resource, 2002. Beauty experts team up to give skin care tips for women of all ages.

Anthony C. Chu and Anne Lovell, *The Good Skin Doctor.* London: HarperCollins, 1999. A dermatologist and an advice columnist team up to discuss the different types of acne, why it occurs, and different conventional and alternative treatments.

Gale Maleskey, *Nature's Medicines.* Emmaus, PA: Rodale Press, 1999. Different herbs, what they do, and what illnesses they treat are discussed in detail.

Linda Papadopoulous and Carl Walker, *Understanding Skin Problems.* West Sussex, England: Wiley, 2003. Provides information and advice on living with different skin conditions, including acne.

Periodicals

Anjana Ahuja, "Could a Jab Cure Teenage Spots?" *Times* (London), November 5, 2001.

Katherine Hobson, "Mind Versus Face," *U.S. News & World Report,* April 1, 2002.

In Style, "Beauty Talk," July 2003.

Joseph A. Witkowski and Lawrence Charles Parish, "Dermatologic Manifestations of Complementary Therapy," *SKINmed,* 2003.

Internet Sources

Acne Net, "Acne Net Update." www.skincarephysicians.com.

Acne.org, "Accutane." www.acne.org.

———, "Success Stories." www.acne.org.

Acne Support Group, "Top Ten Problems." www.stopspots.org.

Australian, "Bleeding Misery of the Boy Cursed by a Common Cure," January 18, 2003. http://searchepnet.com.

American Academy of Dermatology, "Study Confirms Monthly Hormonal Changes in Menstrual Cycle Affect Acne Flare-Ups." www.aad.org.

————, "Study Finds New Laser Treatment Helps Heal the Physical and Emotional Scars of Acne." www.aad.org.

————, "The Social Impact of Acne." www.derm-infonet.com.

Chaos Kids, "Juicy Zits." http://chaoskids.com.

Clare Le Dor.Com, "Clare Lé Dor Natural Acne Treatment System." www.clareledor.com.

Rory Clements, "The Once a Day Gel That Can Beat Acne," *Daily Mail,* (London) March 19, 2002. http://search.epnet.com.

Coenzyme-A Technologies Inc., "Testimonials for Clear Skin Image." www.coenzyme-a.com.

Curelight.com, "CureLight on NBC Health Watch (February 18, 2003). www.curelight.com.

Exposed, "Tips." www.exposedskincare.com.

Hungerstrike.com, "Got Zits?" www.hungerstrike.com.

Marni Leff, "Acne Vaccine May Be on the Horizon," *Seattle Post-Intelligencer,* April 6, 2001. http://seattlepi.nwsource.com.

Julia Necheff, "Emotional Scars from Acne Linger," *Canadian Press,* September 2, 1999. www.slam.ca.

Tamar Nordenberg, "Battling Blemishes and Beyond," Discovery Health Channel. www.health.discovery.com.

Palle Rosted, "Treatment of Skin Diseases with Acupuncture—a Review," The Medical Acupuncture Web Page. http://users.med.auth.gr.

Jennifer Thoden, "How Eight Glasses of Water a Day Can Keep Acne Away," About Holistic Healing. www.healing.about.com.

YM.com, "Newsy Page November 20, 2001. www.ym.com.

Index

see also hormones;
   isotretinoin; treatments
meditation, 47–48
menstruation, 18, 67–69
misconceptions, 6–9, 13

noncomedogenic products, 62,
   64
nutrition, 56, 59–60

oil production
   in adolescents, 17–18
   cortisol and, 20
   environment and, 64
   heat treatments and, 75
   hormones and, 10–12
   isotretinoin and, 31
   menstrual cycle and, 68
   skin cleansing and, 53
   treatment type and, 26–27
   vitamin A and, 29
   vitamin B_5 and, 43
oxidation, 13–14

papules, 13–16, 24–25
perspiration, 59, 64
physical effects, 21–22
phytoestrogen, 40–41, 52
pregnancy, 18–19, 26
progesterone, 21
Propionibacterium acne,
   68–70, 72–74
puberty, 17
pustules, 13–16, 25, 31, 70

rashes, 24
relaxation response therapy,
   46–51
Retin A, 28, 32–33, 38
retinoids, 29–30, 65

Roaccutane. *See* isotretinoin
rosacea, 24
Rosted, Palle, 46

salicylic acid, 26–27, 44
scars
   cystic acne and, 16
   emotional, 22–23
   treatment of, 32, 75–80
   types of, 21–22
seaweed, 44
sebaceous oil glands. *See* oil
   production
sebum
   cortisol and, 48, 57
   excess fat and, 43
   hormones and, 18, 30, 67–68
   isotretinoin and, 31
   overcleansing and, 54
   overdrying and, 64
   production of, 10–14
Shalita, Alan R., 67–68
skin dermabrasion, 26, 32
SKINmed (journal), 52
sleep, 56–58
Smell and Taste Treatment and
   Research Foundation, 51
soaps, 53–55
squeezing, 60–62
stress
   exercise and, 59
   heat-shock proteins and, 70
   hormone levels and, 19–20
   see also treatments
Stupak, Art, 36
sulfur, 28
sunlight, 64–65

tea tree oil, 38, 43
tetracycline, 28–30

Picture Credits

About the Author

Barbara Sheen has been a writer and educator for more than thirty years. She writes in English and Spanish. Her writing has been published in the United States and Europe. She lives in New Mexico with her family, where she enjoys swimming, reading, weight training, and cooking.